The Complete Book of Walking

sets a pace adaptable to every life style. Regardless of age, sex, vocational demands or physical condition, this safe, proven method of walking for your health will change you and your life.

Now, from a team of qualified experts comes the easy and effective Consumer Guide® Walking Program—a tested plan to get you fit and keep you that way!

Learn how the vigorous exercise of walking can strengthen your heart and lungs . . . slow down the aging process . . . relieve stress . . . enhance your figure . . . and add years to your life.

**It's the Natural Way
to Look and Feel Fantastic!**

The Complete Book of Walking

Charles T. Kuntzleman and the Editors of Consumer Guide®

POCKET BOOKS

New York   London   Toronto   Sydney   Tokyo

POCKET BOOKS, a division of Simon & Schuster, Inc.
1230 Avenue of the Americas, New York, N.Y. 10020

Published by arrangement with Publications International Ltd.
Library of Congress Catalog Card Number: 78-78065

ISBN: 0-671-64803-9

First Pocket Books printing March 1982

10 9 8 7

POCKET and colophon are trademarks of
Simon & Schuster, Inc.

Printed in the U.S.A.

CONTENTS

Staying with It   *121*

You want to start walking your way to fitness, but
you're wondering how long you'll be able to maintain your enthusiasm. Here are a few hints on how
to make exercise so convenient and so much fun
that you'll look forward to every walk.

Walk, Weather or Not   *135*

If you succeed in making your walking program as
much a part of your day as eating or sleeping,
you'll probably find yourself walking through
rain, snow, sleet and summer's heat—and enjoying every minute of it.

Some Special Situations   *145*

Heart attack victims, the extremely overweight,
persons with arthritis and emphysema can all
safely engage in a regular program of brisk walking by following our specific guidelines.

Exercises for Walkers   *161*

Walking is the perfect exercise for your heart,
your lungs, your legs and weight control. But it
doesn't do much for your arms, neck or abdomen.
We've put together a series of flexing movements
and calisthenics to help you tone up all over.

Future Generations   *191*

It may seem that children get plenty of exercise.
But their activity probably is not aerobic. Walking
is an outstanding way to get children interested in
their own fitness, and it's something the entire
family can do together.

Walking Tours   *196*

One of the best ways to acquaint yourself with a
city and its people is to walk—either by merely
touring your own hometown or by taking a true
walking vacation to another city. Here are some
recommended tours.

Feats of Walking

Competition almost seems to be a human instinct.
Whatever the endeavor, some people want to do it
best. Among those who have set walking records
are people who've walked across continents,
around the world, even hundreds of miles back-
wards.

FOREWORD:

SOME REMARKABLE PEOPLE.

As you stroll through this book, you're going to meet some remarkable people.

Like Steve McKanic, who, at the age of 46, suffered a severe heart attack and was in a coma for a week. Soon after his attack, he was told by a cardiologist that there was no hope for a coronary bypass operation. He was advised to go home, take his medication, and in effect, wait for the heart attack that would surely kill him. Instead, McKanic quit smoking and started walking. Today, five years later, McKanic is active and optimistic.

There's Elmer Onstott, who carried a heavy back-pack and walked the entire length of the Appalachian Trail, which runs all the way from Georgia to Maine—when he was nearly 70 years old.

Nathalie Smith, racked by tension, had such high blood pressure that her doctor was afraid to let her drive home from his office; he feared she would have a stroke along the way. But she began a program of walking. Now her blood pressure is low, her spirits are high, and *she* is afraid. . . to stop walking.

You'll read about George Hassler Johnson, a man who walked nearly 600 miles in 20 days without eating any food of any kind. You'll find out who holds the world's record for the longest distance walked backward, the youngest person ever to complete the entire Appalachian Trail, and many others.

All of these stories are true. And, though some of them may sound bizarre or frivolous, they are worth considering as you think about your physical condition and the way you live.

Are you convinced that exercise is not beneficial unless it hurts? Are you afraid to try vigorous activity because you have questions about your health? Do you believe that your twice-weekly tennis lessons are keeping you fit? Do you think that dieting is far better than exercising for weight loss because activity makes you hungry? Do you think you're too old or too young to begin a carefully planned walking program?

If you do, you've got another think coming. We're about to give you all the information you need to begin and stay with an exercise program that can add years to your life and life to your years. It can help you lose weight faster than any diet alone. It can improve the efficiency of your heart and lungs, keep you flexible, heighten your awareness, and give you a new sense of confidence in your body.

In the following pages, we'll tell you all about the undeniable benefits of walking, how easy it is to get started, what kind of shoes to wear, how you can measure your success, and where to go on a walking vacation.

The walking program devised by Charles T. Kuntzleman and the editors of CONSUMER GUIDE® is so simple yet so effective that anyone of any age in practically any physical condition can use it.

Some people might call Charles T. Kuntzleman an evangelist, because he preaches the gospel of physical fitness wherever he goes. Kuntzleman, national consultant to the YMCA has worked with the editors of CONSUMER GUIDE® on two previous books: *Rating the Exercises,* and *The Running Book.* He has been running for 25 years and has recommended a running program to many people as a means of getting and staying fit.

However, he says, "Running is not for everyone. For some people it is too strenuous, too demanding. For some it's a hassle. Many people take up running and soon stop. For all these ex-joggers and ex-runners, I submit that walking is the perfect exercise."

In 1974, Kuntzleman was commissioned by Dr. Clayton Myers, director of the Nationwide YMCA Cardiovascular Health Program, to develop two health and fitness programs for the YMCA. The goal of one of these programs was to motivate American adults to exercise—a program that could be taken outside of the YMCA and used in church halls, schools, and apartment complexes all across America. Myers wanted a program that: (1) did not require a lot of sophisticated testing; (2) permitted people to start exercising without having to see their doctor (unless they had a serious question about their health); (3) controlled their body weight; (4) improved their health quotient; (5) reduced selected coronary heart disease risk factors; and (6) improved their fitness level.

Myers said he wanted a program that would keep people exercising. He wanted few or no exercise dropouts.

Kuntzleman concluded that walking was the best exercise for the Y. Everyone can walk: the young and the old; male and female; sick and healthy. So walking became a central theme of Kuntzleman's YMCA Activetics program.

The theory of walking for fitness is one thing; its application is another. So before Kuntzleman released the program to the Y, he tested the concept in the communities of Jackson and Grand Rapids, Michigan, and Allentown, Pennsylvania. The results were amazing. Men and women decreased their weight and body fat, improved their fitness levels, and lowered their blood pressure and their cholesterol levels. Their depression and anxiety seemed to disappear. They felt good about themselves.

Mrs. Kuntzleman, a professional health and physical educator who was teaching at a local college, assisted her husband in his research. She offered classes as a physical fitness and weight control program for adults. Each week, the participants were asked to walk a certain distance. The average person clocked about 30 miles a week. After 15 weeks had elapsed, Mrs. Kuntzleman asked the walkers why they had exercised so faithfully. The list included such comments as: "I feel great," "I sleep better," "No more depression, no more high blood pressure," "I like myself better," "It's fun," "I love life more," and "I have more energy." Over 30 reasons were listed.

Surprisingly, no one mentioned losing weight—although that was the reason why the participants had signed up for the class in the first place. But they did lose weight. Most of them dropped about 10 pounds. However, the weight loss was no longer their only objective. What kept them going was their overall good feeling of well-being. The Kuntzleman's pilot groups of over 300 people included walkers who marked off distances in malls in the Jackson County area so they could keep on walking in the dead of winter.

Kuntzleman and his wife offered a fitness class for couples wherein spouses logged their miles together—the only way they were permitted to record mileage. One week, a man announced that he and his wife had walked 99 miles. Then his wife stood up and said, "But I contributed 66 of them!" There was no shortage of enthusiasm for walking in any of the classes.

It appears that the Kuntzlemans were a bit ahead of their time. When they started the program, it seemed that the only people who walked were those whose cars wouldn't start. But in 1978, at a three-day conference entitled "Exercising and Aging—Its Role In The Prevention Of Physical Decline," held at the National Institute of Health at Bethesda, Maryland, researchers from the United States, Canada, and Western Europe presented papers stating that walking is the most efficient form of exercise, and the only one you can safely follow all the years of your life. We agree wholeheartedly.

It's our goal to make a believer of you, too.

The Complete Book
of Walking

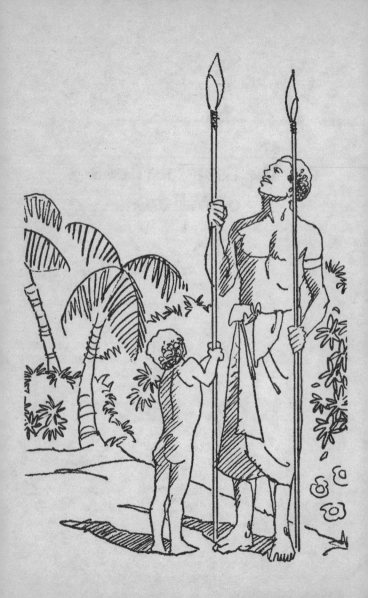

THE PRIMITIVE WAY

WE MAY BE "ADVANCED," BUT THAT DOESN'T MEAN WE'RE FIT.

If you could go back in time and live the way the American pioneers did, would you? Would you trade places with the most isolated bands of Eskimos, whose life is—or used to be—one long, frigid struggle? Can you imagine yourself living as some of the more primitive tribes of Africa do—people whose way of life hasn't changed much since the Stone Age?

Probably not. But if we did go back to the primitive way, we'd be far more fit than we are now. Sophisticated as we members of technologically advanced societies are in our understanding of science and medicine, we can't consider ourselves superior to the primitives in fitness.

Thousands of years ago, walking was the best way or the only way to get around. Today, Australian aborigines still use their feet to secure the basic necessities of life. A group of them stalks a kangaroo mile after mile for days, until the kangaroo is too exhausted to go any further. Then they kill it for food and carry the carcass back the way they came—walking, mile after mile, until they arrive again at their home camp.

Surprisingly, once through the critical period of childhood infectious diseases, the aborigines live as long as the average American, without the help of medical technology.

There are a few other groups of people scattered through the mountain regions of Pakistan, Ecuador, and Russia who have endurance like that of the aborigines. They use their bodies vigorously every day in everything they do. Theirs is a simpler life than we are used to, and it is much more physically active than ours. They eke out an existance that our culture views as primitive, but they live as long—if not longer—than those of us who live in "advanced" societies. These primitive peoples remain active, contributing, vigorous members of their societies right up to death.

Many of these isolated, primitive peoples have little resistance to microbial infections that merely inconvenience us. But they have a much greater resistance to heart disease, diabetes, and the more common forms of cancer—diseases that not only cut life short, but take away enjoyment of life.

Heart disease is the biggest killer of all diseases that plague advanced societies. However, Dr. R. D. Goldrick and his colleagues at the Australian National University found a tribe of natives in New Guinea in which heart disease is extremely rare and diabetes is unknown. Of 777 natives studied, only two had any sign of heart disease.

Goldrick's investigation suggests what other studies on primitive societies have established: the resistance of primitive people to our ailments is not due primarily to genetic immunity, which would be able to protect them even after they began to lead modern lives. It seems certain that their relative freedom from degenerative disease is at least partly due to the fact that life in unmechanized surroundings requires human beings to function near their physical capacity in order to survive. There is growing evidence to support the theory that modern man's failure to use physical powers developed over thousands of years is responsible for his premature physical and mental degeneration.

If you want a specific example of how the sedentary ways of "civilization" offset so-called primitive societies, you have one fairly close to home. This process of physical debilitation has been dramatically documented by researchers studying Eskimos in the Canadian Arctic. In the old days, these hearty people lived a nomadic, self-reliant life. In numbing temperatures of 50 degrees below zero, the men hunted and fished; the women fished through the ice; and walking was always necessary. Now, however, the airplane links Eskimos everywhere with the 20th century. For all but a few of them, walking, driving dog sleds, and living in igloos are only memories. Today's Eskimos drive snowmobiles and live in electrified wooden houses built by the federal government. Once left to die in times of famine, infants and the elderly are now protected by welfare and pensions. But if the Eskimos are further from death than they used to be, they are also further from fitness. The men no longer have to hunt for food. Instead they work at sedentary factory jobs and take their meals in the company cafeteria, where they overeat. The women, who once tanned skins and made their family's clothes, can now purchase their clothing at stores. They have little to do but eat sweets and go to the movies. Bored with the tameness of settlement life, teenagers educated in Bureau of Indian Affairs schools nibble chocolate bars and drink soda pop.

As a result of this sheltered, inactive lifestyle, in one generation the Eskimos have begun to develop degenerative diseases at a frightening rate. Obesity, diabetes, heart disease, and other ailments are starting to weaken bodies that once thrived on the challenge of the frozen North.

It is revealing to compare the sedentary Eskimos with the long-lived people of Hunza in the Himalayas, Ecuador, and Abkhazia in Russia. These people walk everywhere possible. Just scrambling over the slopes of their mountainous homelands has given them a high degree of cardiovascular fitness. Tests by cardiologist David Kaliashvili showed that although these old people have many forms of heart and blood vessel disease, the oxygen supply to their hearts is so good that heart attacks do little harm.

Americans and members of other industrial societies had to work very hard 30, 40, or 50 years ago—so hard that fat was a luxury, a symbol of the leisure class. Most people lived in small towns or on farms, but even city dwellers did a fair amount of walking to work, to market, to visit friends, to parties, to dances. Strolling to and from an evening's entertainment was usually considered part of the entertainment. Getting there was half the fun. Two-story houses were the rule rather than the exception, so most people did a good deal of walking or running up and down stairs.

All this has changed. Modern devices have made us almost completely sedentary. For example, a small thing such as an extension phone in a home saves 70 miles of walking a year. For the average person this means a two-pound weight increase each year. Compare, too, the amount of human energy (calories) spent in using hand tools with the energy expended in using electric models today.

Back in the 1930s, the United States Research Council said that the average sedentary man needed 3,000 calories a day to maintain his body weight; the average woman needed around 2,400. Today, less than 50 years later, the council says a sedentary man requires approximately 2,400 calories a day to maintain that weight and the average female needs as little as 1,800.

Somewhere along the line we've cut 600 calories out of our lives: we burn 600 fewer calories every day. We're great at conserving our own physical energy, but for what purpose? All of this conservation has given us a new problem: obesity. Few people would be happy to go back to the days when everything had to be done by hand or by foot. But our grandparents didn't have to contend with obesity and its related problems.

The trends that encourage obesity are likely to continue. The more labor-saving devices we acquire—and it seems as though someone comes up with a new one every day—the fewer calories we burn away, and the more weight we gain. Inactivity is so much a part of our culture that we actually have to go out of our way to burn off calories. But unless we do, all the energy we're saving by sitting when we should be moving is converted into fat.

When we examine the daily activities of the hardy people who scramble after goats and walk up and down steep hills to gather food or just to bathe in a stream, it becomes clear that in most parts of the world technology has made this kind of vigorous living obsolete. Most of us do not have to walk or do much physical work, either in our occupations or at home. In our present way of life, physical performance is almost unnecessary. The result has been lower vitality. But our scientific sophistication makes us aware that disuse of the body's physical strength is contrary to our evolutionary heritage, and a new concept has emerged. This is *fitness:* the idea that the body's organs and muscles must be exercised regularly if an individual is to preserve a balance between physical and mental development and attain maximum well-being.

There is proof all around us that man should strive to condition his body to be able to bear the stresses of life. Each winter storm kills people who don't realize that shoveling snow can be lethal to the unfit. Sagging and expanding body contours are a constant reminder that lack of movement leads to muscular degeneration. Weakness, shortness of breath, aches and pains, tension and nervousness are common symptoms among today's white-collar workers. All can have their origin in insufficient physical activity. The human mind has achieved remarkable things, but it has yet to create an artificial substitute for exercise.

How can we regain our lost vitality? Do we have to

hunt kangaroos or live in a mountain village and raise goats? No, but we must give our bodies 15 to 60 minutes of activity every day. Leonard A. Larson, former chairman of the Department of Physical Education, Health, and Recreation at the New York University School of Education, says: "The 'key' concept of maintaining good condition is the term consistency, not duration or intensity, although movements must be intense in order to achieve and maintain good physical development." And since walking is so convenient, it should be easy to be consistent.

Nostalgia is very big these days. Tiffany lamps, old Superman comic books, beer cans—anything that reminds us of the good old days is "in." Unfortunately, many Americans aren't nostalgic about the loss of their physical heritage. We need to be more primitive. We've got to get out there and walk.

THE ADVANTAGES
OF WALKING

NOT TOO DIFFICULT, NOT TOO
EASY—WALKING IS JUST RIGHT.

For years, many doctors have said that walking is excellent exercise. We think it's the perfect exercise because almost everyone can walk, without fancy paraphernalia, fees, or instructors. You can fit walking into your particular way of life more easily than almost any other kind of exercise.

Physical fitness experts—such as Dr. Hans Kraus, world famous back specialist; Dr. Theodore G. Klumpp, medical consultant to the President's Council on Physical Fitness and Sports; and Dr. Warren Guild, clinical associate in medicine at Harvard—say walking is an outstanding activity for fitness. Dr. Evelyn S. Gendel, adjunct professor at Kansas University Medical School, has said walking is an "excellent exercise because anyone can do it—in pairs, in groups . . . [it] can be graduated in intensity for any age or physical limitation."

Although not as strenuous as jogging, walking will increase your heart rate and oxygen consumption enough to qualify as an aerobic exercise. An aerobic exercise is the type that gets your whole body, or most of it, moving. It produces a "training effect" on your body by getting your heart to beat fast and your breath to become deep. This is the kind of effect marathon runners experience when they train. Aerobic exercise

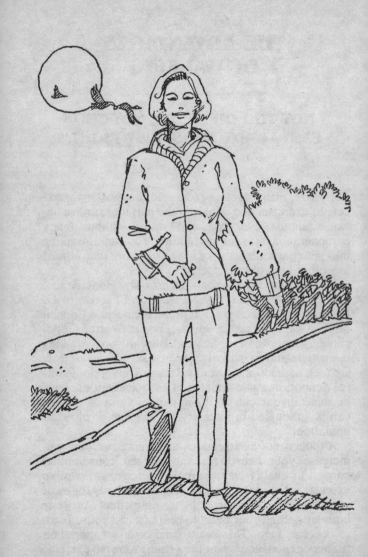

makes your body work better. Most doctors say true health begins with aerobic fitness.

Some people have found out, the hard way, that the use of crash diets and "wonder drugs" for losing weight can be futile or even dangerous. Instead they might have tried walking. Half an hour of vigorous striding burns 180 to 250 calories. A walk like this every day means a weight loss of 15 pounds in a year—without a change of eating habits. Physiologists calculate that 19 percent body fat is ideal for a woman and 15 percent is ideal for a man in terms of overall health. A lower ratio, down to as little as 5 percent fat, is safe and can be desirable for a svelte appearance. Walking can help you maintain a low percentage of body fat.

Walking helps other parts of your body, too. Your digestive system can be made healthier through walking: it stimulates elimination and helps reduce constipation. Walking improves circulation in your legs, which means you can avoid getting varicose veins. Better circulation to your leg muscles can mean less leg fatigue and fewer aches. Walking improves muscle tone in the legs, making them more shapely and healthy-looking. Walking is a natural tranquilizer: it can reduce anxiety and tension. Even depression can be relieved. And walking can lower dynamic blood pressure; that is, your blood pressure under stress.

There are plenty of exercises for which similar claims can be made. However, there is one fact that makes walking best of all for many people: the only exercise that does you any good is the exercise you do; and walking is very easy. It is less demanding than other aerobic exercises like swimming and running. If you're in reasonably good health—free of chest pain, dizziness, and high blood pressure—and if you use good judgment, you shouldn't have any problems. Except in rare cases, you shouldn't need medical clearance, and you certainly won't need the kind of extensive physical exam that is recommended for more strenuous exercise programs. (For safety's sake you should tell your doctor that you're interested in beginning a walking program, but if you use some common sense, you shouldn't have trouble.)

Even heart disease sufferers, the overweight, and people with arthritis and emphysema can enjoy the benefits of walking.

Heart problems induced Casey Conrad to walk for fitness. Conrad, executive director of the President's Council on Physical Fitness and Sports, began walking with his wife as she started a rehabilitation program following a heart valve operation.

Reggie Wright, a walker from Jackson County, Michigan, had started many exercise programs and failed. He always felt he had to jog to get into shape. He became an "exercise dropout." Then about a year ago he decided to try walking. His wife had been extremely successful in losing weight by walking, so he knew it would work. Wright now walks from one to one and a half hours a day. He looks like a different man after having lost over 80 pounds, and he says he feels great.

Walking also can help arthritis victims. Many doctors say walking is the best thing an arthritic can do to slow the spread of the disease, maintain proper body weight, and improve flexibility. Lenny A. Covello, regional associate for the Mid-America Region YMCA, is a good example of what walking can do. He has severe rheumatoid arthritis in his hips. He knows that the disease is progressive; yet he continues to walk. Walking helps him stay limber, and he's able to do more when he is active. His walking program has been approved by his doctors at the Mayo Clinic.

Walking has helped emphysema patients. Several years ago, Dr. Lazlo Ambrus and his co-workers at the Veterans Administration Hospital in Northridge, California, experimented with an exercise program for 43 emphysema patients that included walking. By the end of the study the patients were able to breathe easier, their weight had stabilized, much of their strength had returned, and their endurance had increased. They were able to walk for longer periods of time, from three and a half to more than seven minutes. They breathed easier, literally and figuratively, because they worried less about their condition. They said they enjoyed the program, and even claimed that food tasted better to them. Their outlook on life had improved. Their improved mental state was perhaps the most important result of the study.

Casey Conrad observes: "Walking sharpens your senses. You're able to grasp things, to become more creative. You enjoy the esthetic, grasp the beauty. True vigorous walkers are out looking and thinking in addition to doing. . . . The slogan of walkers is: 'You can't walk away from your troubles but you can sometimes walk them off.'"

Aerobic Capacity: A Test for Fitness

Experts measure a person's fitness in terms of aerobic capacity; that is, the ability to pick up oxygen, send it throughout the body, and use it. This capacity can be measured by an exercise stress test. During such a test, you pedal a stationary bicycle, walk or run on a motorized treadmill, or step on and off a bench—under a doctor's close supervision. Your electrocardiogram is continuously monitored, and your blood pressure is observed to guard against overexertion. At the first sign that the heart is irritated by exercise, the test is stopped. By watching the electrocardiogram, your blood pressure, and your respiration rate, the doctor can tell when you are working to your capacity. The test also involves a measurement of oxygen use. During this part of the test, you breathe into a one-way valve that lets the doctor collect the exhaled air. The air is then analyzed to determine how much oxygen your body used during the activity. The amount of oxygen used represents your aerobic capacity.

Most people do poorly in these tests. It's no wonder, then, that adults completely run out of steam by four or five o'clock in the afternoon. They lack the energy they once had. This is a sign of poor aerobic capacity. Your lungs, heart, blood vessels, and muscles are kept at peak efficiency if you challenge them frequently with regular activity; if you do not, they will start to atrophy or weaken. Their ability to function will be reduced, and you will lose stamina.

Aerobic capacity can be improved by proper walking. When you walk, your heart starts to beat faster and move large amounts of oxygen-rich blood around your body more forcefully. Your blood vessels expand to carry this oxygen. In your working muscles, dormant (unused) blood vessels open up to permit a good pick-up of oxygen and release of carbon dioxide. These changes improve your ability to process oxygen.

Your heart rates during activity and at rest will be reduced greatly. That means your heart will pump more blood with each beat. It's like tuning your car to get more miles to the gallon. The heart of an average adult at rest beats 60 to 80 times a minute. A well-trained heart at rest may beat 40 to 50 times, or even less, a minute. Many people begin an exercise program with a resting heart rate of 80 beats a minute. After three months of walking, it drops to 60; a year later it might stabilize at 50. At that lowest rate, the heart is beating 35,000 fewer times a day than it did before the program began.

At the beginning of a walking program, a person's pulse rate may reach 130 or 140 beats a minute after 20 to 30 minutes of walking. But as weeks go by, the heart becomes more efficient, and the exercise heart rate is lower during the 20 to 30 minutes of walking. To continue enjoying the training effect of walking, the walker must walk faster, or occasionally longer.

Dr. Michael Pollock and his associates explored the importance of different kinds of exercises several years ago. They wanted to find out how walking compared with other forms of exercise, such as jogging, gymnastics, and various athletic games. To do this they chose 16 healthy but sedentary men between the ages of 40 and 56. These men walked from two and a half to three and a half miles each day, four days a week for 20 weeks. As they walked, they tried to keep their heart beat rates within a certain training range. To test the effectiveness of the walking program, the 16 men were tested on a treadmill. While on the treadmill, their oxygen-intake capacities were measured. Their heart rate responses to a standard treadmill walk and to a one-mile walk were also measured. The results: a fast walk can be as effective as a slow jog. The men were able to walk longer at a lower heart beat rate by the end of the 20 weeks. Their oxygen-intake capacity improved. In fact, the researchers said, "The training heart rate data show walking to be a moderate to rigorous activity which has sufficient intensity to cause a significant training effect."

Pollock's group of walkers had to move faster and faster to keep their heart beat rates in the proper range. After the 20 weeks of training, when the men walked at a certain speed on the treadmill, their heart rates were about 17 beats slower than what they were at the beginning of the training program. Pollock's results have been supported by many other studies.

How quickly your heart recovers after exercise is a strong indicator of how fit you are. In Pollock's group, the recovery rates dropped very fast. Recovery heart rates at one, three, and five minutes after exercise were about 19 to 24 beats per minute slower than when the program began. In other words, Pollock's 16 subjects experienced the training effect, which shows that walking is excellent for building stamina and endurance. That's why walking helps you overcome late afternoon fatigue.

You can start a walking program as you would another type of exercise regimen, setting aside a specific time of time, buying yourself a special walking outfit, joining or forming a walking club. Or you can work it into your present life style so gradually that walking will not noticeably interfere with anything else you do.

Dr. Irving Wright, a cardiologist and clinical professor emeritus at Cornell University, tells his patients to get off the subway two exits early and walk the rest of the way. The doctor follows his own prescription, for he often walks down 15 flights of stairs from high in a New York hospital instead of riding the elevator.

One corporate executive has found a way to make good use of layover time between airplanes. If she has a two-hour wait between flights, she rents a locker in the airport terminal. She takes off her street shoes and puts on her hiking shoes. Then she puts the rest of her belongings in the locker and takes off for a walk around the terminal. She sees all sorts of interesting sights and enjoys herself immensely—more than most people do during a layover or a flight delay. And all the while she is improving her good health and trim figure.

Walking Is for Men and Women

We hope you agree with the statement above, and we hope you're wondering why we felt we had to say so. Unfortunately, some women avoid rigorous physical exercise because of a socialized bias against it, and some men believe walking is not strenuous enough to have a significant effect on fitness. The truth is walking can be beneficial to men and women, because the fitness needs of the two sexes are nearly identical.

Research done by Dr. Jack Wilmore shows that—except for upper body strength, lean body weight, and height—there is little difference in the overall strength, endurance and body composition of male and female athletes. And, although the female may weigh less than the male, the ratio of fat to overall weight of physically fit men and women is just about the same. Wilmore says, "Because of these similarities, and because their needs are essentially the same, there is little reason to advocate different training or conditioning programs on the basis of sex."

Women have different fitness needs only in the sense that they need exercise even more than men: the average woman is less fit than the average man. The reason is cultural, not biological. American cultural patterns—and even some exercise experts—tend to overprotect women and discourage them from physical activity after puberty. Over the years, popular culture has prized a shapely female figure; yet it has also perpetuated the myth that exercise is unfeminine. The fact is that exercise is a necessity for women who want to develop and maintain attractive bodies.

Times are changing, and that's good. Research has clearly demonstrated the value of exercise in good health and beauty, so increasing numbers of young women are exercising. But cultural biases against vigorous exercise still exist, especially among women past 35. Many of these women like walking because it is "safe" and socially nonthreatening. There probably are four reasons why walking is a great way for women to ease into exercise: they don't have to be proficient at athletics; they can combine walking with other activities and therefore work a walking program into a busy schedule; no special clothing is needed; and walking is a low-sweat exercise.

Take a look at any of the leading women's magazines. Chances are, you'll see photographs of women running, bicycling, or playing tennis; but they never, never seem to work up a sweat. Some women remain convinced that exercise will ruin their hair, soak their clothes, run their mascara and enlarge their calves to unattractive proportions. Even if this were true, the effects of a lack of exercise are far worse.

Many women who today do not like to exercise feel the way they do because they were excused from physical education in high school for a lot of silly reasons. Overprotective parents and doctors, and misinformed physical education teachers deprived girls and young women of the early training that would have inspired them to keep fit.

Walking can change all of this. Once women start walking, they begin to feel better mentally and physically, so they develop an interest in doing other physical things. Many women have become avid runners, tennis players, golfers, and squash and racquetball players after taking up walking. The walking helped them become physical beings. And suddenly many of them discover that migraine headaches, menstrual discomforts, depression and other problems diminish or disappear. The walking also improves their appearance, so their self-concept improves. Now they feel good about themselves, and see clearly that exercising is the right thing to do. Walking has liberated them from restrictive attitudes. They are now ready for increased activity. If they'd tried swimming or tennis as an initial activity, some of these women would have quit after a few sessions. But walking succeeded in pulling them into a more active life style. Today's modern woman understands that motion is important in her life. If she wants to live her life to the fullest, she needs to exercise.

Men have a problem with sweat, too. Only this time it is the reverse. Many men think the only good exercise is exercise that hurts and makes them sweat like a horse. Consequently, some men play basketball once a week in rubberized sweatsuits. They certainly do sweat a lot, and they think that will keep them fit. In fact, however, they're headed for heart, muscle, and joint trouble.

Some men run for fitness. That's fine. But what isn't

fine are judgmental statements such as, "girls walk; running is for men." That attitude stems from a man's younger days. When in school, many boys run to get into shape. They run wind sprints at the end of the sports practice and more laps when disciplined. Unlike women, men are expected to run in their teenage years.

This is good training for performance. It makes sense. But we're concerned with fitness, not sports. Fitness means improved heart-lung function that will help you get through the day without excessive fatigue. Fitness means control of your body weight. It also implies reducing the risk of coronary heart disease and making you feel better. In other words, the goal of fitness is to help you achieve better health and well-being. Unfortunately, many men think fitness and sports are synonymous.

For all these reasons, men think running is far better than walking to get into shape. So they run. But soon many of them grow to dislike it. They remember the wind sprints, the laps, and all the other distasteful things about high school sports and never get around to exercising on a permanent basis. They know they need exercise. They talk about it, but they don't want to get involved and be committed to it. Instead, they play their basketball once a week and expect that to do the job. It won't. This is most unfortunate and can be disastrous. The story of a fellow we'll call Bill is a good example.

Bill's wife, Sandy, started to walk for physical fitness. She averaged about 60 to 80 minutes of walking a day for a year. Sandy tried to get Bill to walk off some pounds (he weighed 300). Occasionally he did walk. One day a friend saw the two walking together. Trying to encourage them, he called and said: "Hey, that's neat. The two of you walking together—keep it up." What did Bill say? "Ah, this walking isn't any good. Sandy walks too slow and I always have to wait for her. I want to run." Sandy could have walked circles around Bill any day of the week, but Bill had a difficult time admitting it. And as things turned out, Bill wound up with more than wounded pride. Bill showed up at a two-mile "fun run" in his community. Participants were given the choice of walking or running. Of course, Bill decided he was going to run, since everyone would be watching. He ran the distance. He also collapsed at the finish line and had to be hospitalized.

The important ingredient in fitness is how consistently, not how hard, you work. Running is a super way to get fit. So is bicycling and swimming—if you do it regularly and approach it in a sane manner. But many men don't. The best way to start a fitness program is by walking. Take your time and see what happens.

Doug Race, Director of Developmental Education at Jackson Community College in Jackson, Michigan, was having some orthopedic problems four years ago. After his foot operation, he looked at his feet and didn't like what he saw. He decided to get up and do something about it. He started walking while still in the hospital. Before he came home, he was able to do two miles a day painlessly on carpet. Little by little he added distance or time—six miles; eight; then 10. At one point, he was doing as much as 80 or 90 miles a week. Then he felt he was strong enough to turn to running. Today if he does 10 miles, he'll walk five and run the other five.

Race sometimes walks for distance, sometimes for time, depending on how he feels on a particular day. "I walk the halls early in the morning at work. I'm alone with nothing to bother me. It gets my mind together for the day." Each morning he tries to walk at least two miles. He'll also walk at noon and again in the evening. He has built walking into his daily routine. His advice to men who are thinking about walking is very simple: "Just begin with a good shoe and walk no farther or faster than you feel comfortable. And then little by little you can treat walking like you do running. You can speed train, or you can distance train. You can vary the distance and speed and you can play with it. It's like a game. You can go hard one day and light the next. Little by little build up. If you do reach a point sometime when you want to run, then I think you're ready for it. But quite frankly, I don't think any man should give up the joy of walking."

Nor should women. Nor should people of either sex who have specific physical problems. They shouldn't allow themselves to believe that they can't benefit from walking. Walking is for everybody.

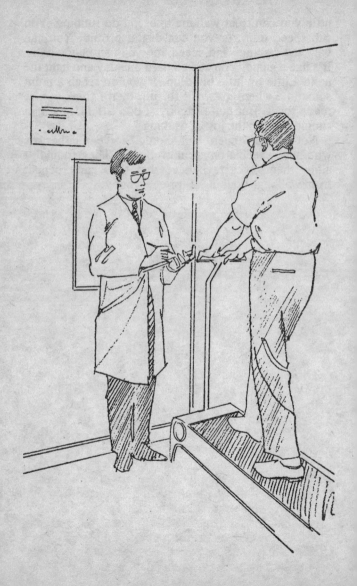

WALKING FOR YOUR HEART

STUDIES SHOW THAT YOU CAN AVERT ATTACKS AND REPAIR DAMAGE.

Steve McKanic, of Concord, Michigan, had a severe heart attack in May 1973. He spent two weeks in intensive care. It was touch and go: during the first week he was in a coma most of the time.

After a month's hospitalization, he was sent home under the care of his family physician. In July he was referred to a cardiologist in Kalamazoo, who tested him to find out whether McKanic could be helped by coronary bypass surgery. The doctor's conclusion was:

The work up on this gentleman showed almost terminal coronary heart disease. He has reached the stage that is now being called "ischemic cardiomyopathy" of a severe degree and I believe we are not going to be able to help him through surgical bypass of his stenosis. . . . I believe that the treatment at present should include Digitalis preparation, diuretic therapy, a low salt diet and long periods of absolute rest. He may have to lose weight to achieve a more normal pattern. . . . I am very sorry that I am unable to give you better news regarding his future but perhaps it may be possible to keep this patient comfortable for some time to come with the preceding therapy.

In short, McKanic's condition was "hopeless." He was told to go home, get his things in order, and wait for the Big One. To help him manage his heart disease, he was given four types of medication: a vessel dilator, a tranquilizer, and two heart regulators. He was also instructed not to do anything physical.

After the typical period of mental depression, McKanic decided to do something about his health. He sold his four businesses, stopped smoking four packs of cigarettes a day, changed his diet drastically to try to lose weight, and started walking. "Intuitively I knew I should start to move. It just seemed like the thing to do," he says. He also decided to think positively about his health and life in general.

McKanic didn't make these changes overnight. As he read and learned more about his condition, he made gradual adjustments in his life style. For example, when he walked he would go to the point of pain (about one block). He walked at night so no one would see him, because people near to him were convinced he would kill himself. "Many well-intentioned people treated me like a freak," he says. As his condition improved, he walked farther and farther—up to three or four miles a day. His weight dropped from 240 to 164 pounds.

In the meantime, he was placed on 100 percent disability. About 10 months after that happened, the Veterans Administration asked him to go to its hospital in Ann Arbor. The VA wanted to check McKanic to make sure the disability report was justified. After examining him thoroughly, VA officials told him to go home, bide his time, take his medicine, and not engage in any physical activity—sex included.

It was at this point that McKanic said no. He told the doctor, "I'm going to outlive you." He went home, threw his medicine away, and enthusiastically pursued his new life style. In short, he said he had had enough of negative thinking. "No one could get well with that attitude," he told us. So he refused to visit any other doctors.

Today, McKanic is a vibrant, vigorous man of 51. Optimistic about life and his condition, he covers nine to 10 miles a day—without fail. He wasn't an expert; he didn't have a research team; he didn't have a college education. Yet on his own he wrote himself a prescription that has worked for him.

McKanic wanted to learn more. So in January 1978 he enrolled in an exercise class at a local college. When his teacher heard about his physical condition, she was shocked. But she realized McKanic was serious and would continue to exercise with or without her help. She told McKanic about the importance of warm-up and cool-down periods, she told him why he should avoid lifting weights, and she cautioned him on his intensity of exercise (he was jogging at the time). But he replied, "Don't worry about me. I know how to listen to my body."

McKanic's mind and body seem to be right in tune. In June 1978, he decided to go to Canada and take care of a hernia that had plagued him for the previous five years. Why did he pick that particular hospital in Canada? He'd heard you could walk to and from the operating room. So McKanic walked to the operating room, underwent a 50-minute hernia operation, and walked back. Then he got up and walked around the floor for the rest of the day, which was Friday. On Saturday and Sunday he walked more. He even went outside. On Monday morning McKanic was discharged and drove home—an eight-hour drive.

McKanic is in tune with life in general. He has a small business he loves. He is an exciting person to be around. Doctors would like to examine him. We think it would be a good idea, and we've told him so. But his answer is "No. Doctors are too negative. To live you must think positively. That way you can really live and enjoy life." Considering his success, his prescription is difficult to refute. McKanic could still have another heart attack, and he knows it. But he says, "I've just begun to live. My new life style of positive thinking, good fuel for my body, and walking have given me a new life—a life the doctors couldn't and wouldn't give me."

We want to emphasize as strongly as we possibly can that we are not advocating McKanic's program. He has taken some big chances with his life. He could have been wrong in throwing away his pills, in giving up on doctors. Then his story wouldn't have appeared in this book.

We also want to state that walking alone cannot be credited with McKanic's remarkable recovery. The factors that lead to heart ailments and the means by which heart patients regain their health are so poorly understood that it would be irresponsible for us or anyone else to recommend McKanic's approach. Yet he can be admired and respected for his determination and his pursuit of an exercise program that seems to have extended his life.

Adding Years to Your Life.

Many people refuse to believe that exercise will lead to a longer life. They point to statistics that seem to show that, although Americans are becoming increasingly sedentary, they are living longer.

However, when the United States is compared with all of the world's other countries in terms of longevity, the U.S. doesn't measure up: the American male ranks 22nd and the American female ranks 10th. Recent statistics show that the U.S. ranks 37th in life expectancy for men 40 years of age. Twenty years ago, we were 11th. Today, an American boy or girl may have a life expectancy of around 66 and 71 years of age. That appears to be a significant improvement over the life expectancy as calculated in 1900: around 47 to 49 years. But these figures are deceptive. The life expectancy figures do not give the actual age when most people die. Instead, the figures simply tell you the average age of death when you lump all the ages together. In those countries that have a high infant death rate, the average life expectancy is quite low. It is low even though many people live to an advanced age. But when medicine can save the lives of small children, life expectancy figures for the entire population soar.

This is why our life expectancy appears to have risen over the years. Until the 1850s, only half the children born in the U.S. reached the age of five. Today, almost 98 percent make it to that age. That fact is bound to pull up our life expectancy. In 1790, a 60-year-old veteran of the American Revolution had a life expectancy of about 15 more years. Incredibly, his 60-year-old counterpart today has almost the same number of years to live. So it appears that even though we are increasing our longevity as a nation, individuals in America are not living longer than they did 100 or 200 years ago.

The reason why we are not living longer is that degenerative diseases (particularly heart disease) are cutting our lives short. What is especially depressing is that these degenerative diseases also rob us of the "good life." We're tired before the end of the day. Walking is an effort. Life has no joy. Things are too much of a hassle. Our productivity is curtailed. Many of us are not running on all of our cylinders because we suffer from one or more of these modern plagues.

We think exercise can reverse this process. Some critics may say that there is not enough evidence to prove that all people who exercise live longer than people who don't. That is so. But on the other hand, research has not been able to prove the contrary. And while there are many variables regarding exercise and longevity, research is starting to move closer to definite conclusions.

Dr. Charles L. Rose and his associates at the Veterans Administration Outpatient Clinic of Boston explored the relationship between exercise and longevity. The researchers interviewed close relatives of 500 men who died in Boston in 1965. They asked many questions about smoking, eating, exercise, sleeping, recreation, and occupational habits—more than 200 factors. The researchers then arranged the data, looking for interactions of these factors relative to longevity. The results were fascinating: (1) physical exertion during leisure hours benefited people more than exertion on the job; and (2) physical exertion off the job, particularly during the years 40 to 49, were among the best of all longevity predictors. It has been estimated that coronary heart disease robs the average American of seven to 11 years of life. In other words, if coronary heart disease were eliminated, the average American would live seven to 11 years longer than he or she does now.

A large-scale health survey based on a study of 7,000 adults in California over a long period of time demonstrated an 11.5-year greater life expectancy for people whose life styles incorporated six or seven basic health requirements versus those with three or fewer of them. You've probably already guessed the factors. They were: (1) moderate, regular exercise; (2) normal weight; (3) breakfast every day; (4) regular meals with no snacks in between; (5) seven or eight hours of sleep per night; (6) moderate drinking (one small drink or less daily); and (7) no smoking. The findings of this California study were duplicated in a Wisconsin study on 2,000 people.

A few of you may protest. You might say, "I know a guy who exercised regularly every day of his life and he died of a heart attack at 46." But that is a function of heredity. No one can guarantee that if you "live right" you will live longer than your sedentary brethren. If you exercise, you'll get closer to your potential for old age; yet you may not live longer than your sedentary neighbor. Sound contradictory? It isn't. Here's why.

The latest research seems to indicate that we inherit our parents' potential for longevity and fitness. Then our circumstances and the choices we make each day chop months or years away from that allotted life span and influence the degree of our fitness and longevity. For example, although genetically your parents may have had the capacity to live to be 100, perhaps their circumstances and their habits caused them to die much earlier than that. Likewise, although you may have inherited the capacity to live to be 100, your environment and your habits—many of which are learned from your parents—may enable you to live only to the age of 65 or 70. What's more, if you live in noisy, polluted surroundings and do "head work" all day long, forgetting to exercise your senses, your muscles, and your organs, you will forfeit your potential for fitness and longevity.

The Specter of Heart Disease

Coronary artery disease is responsible for the deaths of almost 700,000 people in this country every year. It has been estimated that 12 million Americans are currently being treated for heart disease; another 12 million have it and don't know it. This high rate of coronary disease is largely responsible for the relatively poor life expectancy rate of males in the United States.

If over 10 percent of the population were to come down with some kind of exotic virus or flu, there would be great public uproar. Yet we accept coronary heart disease as an inevitable occurrence, just one of those things: pimples at 13, a coronary at 50. This is a real tragedy, for some cardiologists feel that heart disease can be prevented or postponed so that it won't occur before the age of 70.

Heart disease is a complicated ailment. Many factors are involved, including body weight, diet, activity, blood fats, and others. It is important to remember that walking is just one limited part of treating this disease. Fitness, like medicine, is not a magic cure-all in its effects on the human circulatory system.

The circulatory system includes the heart, arteries, veins, and capillaries. This system circulates blood to all parts of your body. The blood provides body tissues with oxygen and food, and removes waste.

The heart is made of muscle tissue called the myocardium. Like all muscles, the heart must have a continuous blood supply. But blood doesn't simply rush through the heart. It is sent through a special set of arteries, the coronary arteries, which surround the myocardium.

Human beings have a unique need for a "second heart." Four-legged animals don't need such a second heart because all their vital organs are on the same level. The heart, brain, lungs, and even the reproductive glands of four-legged creatures have an easy time getting all the blood they need. But human beings stand upright, so the human circulatory system has to cope with gravity. Nature had to devise a way to pump the blood straight up. The muscles around the veins are pressed into service. Muscles in your feet, calves, thighs, buttocks, and abdomen compose this second heart. As they work, they rhythmically contract and release, squeezing the veins and forcing the blood along, easing the load of pushing 72,000 quarts of blood through your system every 24 hours through nearly 100,000 miles of circulatory byways. It's nature's way of moving the blood to the heart despite the pull of gravity. These second heart muscles work best when you walk.

The key to the efficiency of the circulatory system is walking. Walking makes the muscles below the waist do their part in helping the heart. Without this help, there can be unhappy consequences sometimes, like varicosities or phlebitis. The heart must work harder when it doesn't get assistance from your leg muscles.

For this reason, (and many others) walking has become important in the treatment of heart patients. Doctors now know that walking is the best way to make the lower muscles do their share of the work and relieve a damaged heart. Even a little walking improves circulation and costs the heart no effort. Surprisingly, people whose heart rate and blood pressure are high will find that daily walking helps bring the heart rate and blood pressure down to more normal levels.

A heart attack is not primarily a disease of the heart muscle, but of the arteries that supply the heart muscle with blood. The heart, just like any other muscle, receives its blood supply from the arteries that run through it.

In the anatomy of the human heart, an extensive network of arteries grows out from two main trunks, the right and left coronary arteries. These branch out much like a tree. Each branch is smaller than the main trunk, and each one subdivides into smaller branches. Those in turn divide into still smaller ones, like tiny twigs. Every part of the heart, no matter how small, is supplied with blood and oxygen through the system of coronary arteries, vessels, and capillaries.

In order to understand coronary heart disease, it is important to become familiar with the following terms.

Arteriosclerosis: a general term for various types of arterial illness. The phrase, "hardening of the arteries" is often used for arteriosclerosis. It is associated with a gradually increasing brittleness of arteries.

Atherosclerosis: slowly developing disease of the coronary arteries. In atherosclerosis, the passageway through the arteries becomes roughened and narrowed by fatty deposits that harden into patches along the inner lining of the artery. Consequently, the channel is gradually narrowed, and there is less room for blood to flow through.

Coronary occlusion: a severe narrowing of some coronary artery to the point that blood can no longer pass through.

Coronary thrombosis: a coronary occlusion caused by the formation of a blood clot (thrombus) that completely blocks the flow of blood to some part of the heart muscle.

Myocardial infarction: a condition in which the blood supply to a portion of the muscle is blocked, causing the muscle fed by the blocked artery to die.

Loafer's Heart: a term coined by Dr. Wilhelm Raab, professor emeritus of the University of Vermont College of Medicine, to describe the weakening of the heart muscle as a result of a lack of exercise. It is not the so-called athlete's heart, which should not be considered abnormal for that is a strong and well-developed heart, but the degenerated, inadequate loafer's heart that is a cause for concern.

Collateral circulation: the opening of new arteries and the growth of new branches to offset the effects of atherosclerosis. It is fortunate that the coronary system is able to grow and repair itself. When some of the coronary arteries become narrowed by gradual development of atherosclerosis, nearby arteries get wider and even open up tiny new branches to bring blood to the area of the heart that needs it. Collateral circulation explains why many people who have a narrow artery do not suffer heart attacks and also accounts for some of the excellent recoveries from attacks. Steve McKanic may be a good example of how collateral circulation allows for such recoveries.

Benefits of Exercise

Hundreds of studies have been conducted worldwide to determine why so many people develop heart disease. The causes remain very much a mystery, although many researchers believe they've found a relationship between exercise and healthy hearts. It seems that people who are very active are less likely to suffer heart disease than people who seldom exercise.

A study of two groups of adults in Switzerland showed the relationship between heart disease and lack of exercise. One group was from a mountain village called Blattendorf. These people were compared with a similar group of adults who lived in the town of Basel. The residents of Blattendorf lived several miles from the nearest cart path. So the mountain villagers had to walk everywhere. Climbing mountains and carrying heavy loads were part of their daily routine. They had a much lower percentage of heart disease than did the sedentary inhabitants of Basel, who did very little walking. Studies from all over the world have supported the findings of the Swiss study. In the early 1950s, the health records of 31,000 double-decker bus workers in London were studied. The active conductors who frequently walked around the bus and climbed the stairs were found to have a lower mortality rate and a remarkably faster recovery rate from heart attacks than did the inactive bus drivers.

In 1973, a group of doctors did a different kind of study. Instead of comparing the incidence of heart disease among people in physically active and inactive occupations, the researchers studied the amount of leisure-time exercise in which the people were involved. All aspects of their life style, except for the amount of exercise they got, were the same. The report of the study speaks for itself: "eleven percent of the men who developed coronary disease, compared with twenty-six percent of the controls, reported vigorous activity. In men recording vigorous exercise, the relative risk of developing coronary disease was about a third that in comparable men who did not, and in men reporting much of it still less. Vigorous exercise apparently protected against rapid fatal heart attacks and other first clinical attacks of coronary disease alike, throughout middle age."

Exactly how strong is the relationship between heart disease and inactivity? In 1977, Dr. Ralph Paffenbarger, professor of epidemiology at Stanford University of Medicine, reported on a 10-year study that focused on 17,000 Harvard alumni men aged 35 to 74. He was quite specific: those who burned up less than 2,000 calories a week in exercise were 64 percent more likely to suffer a heart attack than those who burned more than that. Of the 572 heart attacks suffered by the group, he estimated that 166 would never have happened if the men had exercised vigorously. And Paffenbarger said it didn't really matter what kind of exercise was performed, provided the exercise placed a demand on the heart. Golf, bowling, and archery did not qualify, but walking, jogging, swimming, and other demanding activities did.

A recent meeting of scientists in New York City addressed itself to marathon running. At that meeting, the experts concluded that people who adopted the life style of a marathon runner (who is able to run 26.2 miles nonstop, train 36-plus miles a week, and does not smoke) had very little likelihood of developing a coronary. One physician, Dr. Thomas Bassler, a pathologist in Inglewood, California, went so far as to say that this type of life style provides *immunity* from coronary artery disease. Many doctors, including the scientists at that New York meeting, would shy away from Bassler's statement. But one thing is clear: a marathoner's way of life would greatly reduce your chances of having a heart attack.

Why Does Walking Work?

Walking can reduce *many* of your risk factors—those things that increase your chances of getting a heart attack—not just one. There are 11 factors that affect your chances of getting coronary heart disease: heredity, stress, diet, fat abnormalities, hypertension, heart beat abnormalities, diabetes, obesity, smoking, age, and lack of physical activity. Of these 11, walking may improve all except age and heredity. Of course, smoking and diet are not altered by walking itself. Usually, however, people who walk on a regular basis adopt more healthful life styles. They often stop smoking, or cut back substantially, and start eating less. They also tend to eat wholesome foods, because they become more in tune with their bodies.

A recent study by Dr. Kenneth Cooper, author of *Aerobics,* demonstrated the connection between a person's level of aerobic capacity and selected coronary heart disease risk factors. The conclusion was unavoidable: as a person's fitness level improves, his coronary heart disease risk factors drop substantially. The heart disease risk factors affected were cholesterol, triglycerides, glucose, uric acid, systolic blood pressure, and body fat measurements. Men of very poor or poor aerobic fitness showed poor results; those of fair aerobic fitness appeared to be less prone to heart ailments than those in the very poor or poor categories. But they were not as good as those in the excellent category. Those people who scored good and excellent on the aerobic fitness test had the lowest scores on the selected heart disease risk factors. Cooper's study involved 2,998 men with an average age of 44.6 years. To Cooper, it didn't matter which aerobic activity was used for fitness as long as the men got enough exercise to move into the good or excellent fitness category.

Although it is clear that walking helps the heart, blood, and blood vessels, no one knows exactly why. Dr. Samuel Fox, past president of the American College of Cardiology, has several theories. He feels that aerobic exercise (including walking) may:

1. Increase the number and size of your blood vessels for better and more efficient circulation.
2. Increase the elasticity of the blood vessels and thereby reduce the likelihood of their breaking under pressure.
3. Increase the efficiency of exercising muscles and blood circulation so that muscles and blood are better able to pick up, carry, and use oxygen.
4. Increase the efficiency of the heart, making it able to pump more blood with fewer beats and better able to handle emergencies.
5. Increase tolerance to stress and give you more joy of living, which means you will be less likely to be caught in the stress/pressure syndrome.
6. Decrease triglyceride (fats) and cholesterol levels so as to reduce the likelihood of fats being deposited on the lining of the arteries.
7. Decrease clot formation so there is a smaller chance of a blood clot forming and blocking blood flow to the heart muscle.
8. Decrease blood sugar, reducing chances of blood sugar being changed into triglycerides.
9. Decrease obesity and high blood pressure, which is good since most people who are obese and have high blood pressure are more prone to heart disease.
10. Decrease hormone production—good because too much adrenalin can cause problems for the arteries.

Of all the reasons Fox mentioned, the most controversial has been No. 6; that is, that exercise will decrease triglyceride and cholesterol levels. Perhaps no other area has been subject to more controversy.

Doctors now know that it's not the quantity of cholesterol that's important, but how the cholesterol is carried. In your bloodstream, cholesterol is contained within several different types of large conglomerates of proteins and fatty substances. Surprisingly, cholesterol only misbehaves when it falls in with the wrong crowd.

A cholesterol molecule that is bound up with a high-density lipoprotein (HDL) is probably on its way back to the liver to be excreted back into the intestinal tract and eliminated from the body. Cholesterol carried by a low-density lipoprotein (LDL), on the other hand, is meant to be taken up by the body cells as a building block for hormones and cell membranes. Although this lipoprotein is necessary, when there is too much of it in the blood it is not good. Some of it will probably help build up atherosclerotic plaques on the insides of arteries.

Scientists theorize that HDL cholesterol can actually interfere with the process of atherosclerosis. The HDLs may pick up the extra cholesterol in the body and take it back to the liver for removal from the body. A high amount of HDL and a low level of LDL seems to offer some insurance against atherosclerosis. People with low levels of HDL cholesterol have eight times the rate of heart disease as those with higher levels. Fewer LDLs means there is less likelihood of the cholesterol being deposited on the lining of the arteries; more HDLs means more cholesterol is carried for removal from the body.

It now appears that regular, vigorous exercise is helpful in providing a desirable HDL-LDL ratio. Studies show that people who participate in an aerobic-type exercise program for 30 to 45 minutes four times a week find that their HDL levels begin to climb after only seven to 10 weeks.

Another controversial area is the effect of exercise on high blood pressure. Although many doctors now use walking as an adjunct to hypertension therapy, disagreement is everywhere.

One area in which there is little disagreement is the

effect of walking on your dynamic blood pressure. Your dynamic blood pressure is a measure of your blood pressure throughout the day, not just the reading you get at the doctor's office. Your blood pressure can drop or climb throughout the day. During relaxing moments it is probably low; when you're feeling stress, it may zoom upward. Many doctors now feel that the real benefit of exercise is that it helps modulate your dynamic blood pressure. You'll still have valleys and peaks, for you're still subjected to pressures throughout the day. But exercise, such as walking, will see to it that the peaks are not as high as they used to be.

How much exercise do you need to enjoy the 10 positive changes that Fox mentioned as by-products of aerobic exercise? How much exercise do you need to have a good HDL-LDL ratio? And how much exercise do you need to keep your dynamic blood pressure from fluctuating too much?

Doctors are still trying to successfully answer these complex questions. But 45 minutes or more of walking at your target heart rate, four times a week, seems to do it for most people. Yet walking is not a panacea for heart disease. You may have to make other modifications in your living pattern to reduce your risk factors. Select foods carefully; deal with stress in a positive manner; don't smoke.

Recent statistics released by the National Institute of Health show that the incidence of fatal heart disease has decreased by about 14 percent among Americans over the past 20 years. Three reasons given for this drop are better dietary habits, less smoking, and more exercise. Significantly, the most important change was that exercise habits improved.

Walking is a positive approach to better quality of life and health. Walking is something you can actually look forward to; not something to avoid. You don't go to movies you dislike, you don't read books that are boring, you select your friends with care. So why pick an exercise program you won't like?

WALKING TO LOSE WEIGHT

WALKING AND DIETING ARE BETTER THAN DIETING ALONE.

It's not difficult to find so-called weight control experts who doubt the effectiveness of exercise as a method of weight reduction. They hold two misconceptions. First, they say exercise demands relatively little caloric expenditure and is therefore innefficient; and second, they believe exercise increases the appetite and is self-defeating as a weight control method.

Let's look at the first misconception. The body maintains a fine balance between the number of calories taken in and the number of calories burned up through physical activity. For example, if a person takes in 2,400 calories of food and burns up 2,400 calories during sleeping, eating, working, walking, etc., he will maintain his present body weight. But if he eats 2,400 calories in a day and burns up only 2,300, he will have 100 calories left over. Those excess calories will then be stored as fat in the fat cells in the body until they are needed.

Physiologists tell us that approximately 3,500 calories equal one pound of fat. It doesn't matter what type of food is eaten—nutritious food or "junk"—it all contains calories, and they all count. So if 100 calories remain unburned at the end of each day for 35 days, the body will gain one pound of fat. By the end of a year, the body will have gained 10 pounds at that rate. This is the cumulative nature of weight gain.

This sort of slow gain that most people experience

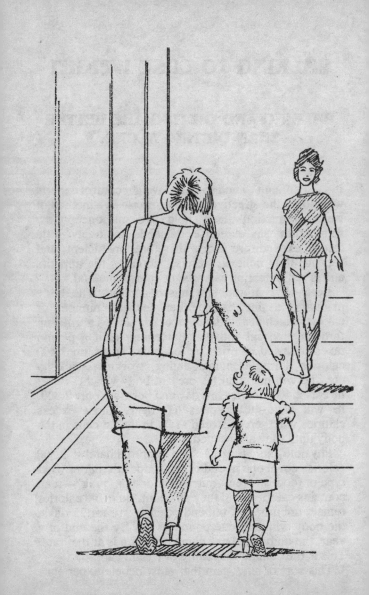

has been called "creeping obesity." Usually, weight gain is noticed over a period of months or years, not overnight. One year you buy a 36-inch belt; the next year you need a 38-inch one.

Walking can be used to turn this process around— sort of a beneficial "creeping fat loss." At your brisk walking speed, you may have to walk for 12 hours to burn up one pound of fat, but it need not be done in a single 12-hour period. Half an hour of walking every day can result in a 15-pound weight loss each year. Extend each walk to an hour, and you can expect to lose 30 pounds. Many times, a 30-minute walk each day is all you need to get yourself back into caloric balance and then start losing weight.

Does this seem to be an exaggeration? Again, we'll let the facts speak for themselves. Time and motion studies have shown that the average overweight person walks about 2.2 miles a day; a person of average build walks 4.8 miles a day. The difference of 2.6 miles is the caloric equivalent of 200 to 300 calories a day— 20 to 30 pounds a year.

Now for the second misconception: the belief that an increase in physical activity is a self-defeating weight control method because it increases appetite. Exercise does indeed increase the appetite of normally active people. This is one of the body's protective mechanisms. Without it, the body of a person who walks an hour extra each day, thereby expending the caloric equivalent of 30 pounds a year, obviously would burn away to nothing over a period of four or five years. The increase in hunger makes it possible to exercise without undermining well-being.

However, the principle does not work in reverse. If you decrease your activity below a moderate level, you will not decrease your appetite. In fact, your appetite will probably increase with inactivity. For many people, eating is a nervous habit. It's something they do just to keep their hands busy. When they're watching TV, sitting is not enough. They seem to like to have a beverage in one hand and potato chips or pretzels in another. Of if they go to a coffee klatch, it's a natural thing to be balancing a sweet roll and a cup of coffee (laced with sugar and cream) on their laps. When you are just sitting around doing next to nothing, you tend to eat more.

Observations of laboratory animals and human beings support this. While professor of nutrition at Harvard University, Jean Mayer and some of his colleagues studied the relationship between food intake, exercise, and weight in white mice. The result: the sedentary mice ate more than the moderately active group and slowly gained weight. The mice that exercised most ate more than the moderately active group, but they had the lowest weight of all the mice. The moderately active mice ate less than the other two groups. Their weight was right in the middle, halfway between the sedentary mice and the very active mice. Another study by Mayer showed that the same thing is true for human beings. His study of overweight high-school girls indicated that they ate no more and some ate less than their normal-weight classmates. However, the overweight girls exercised far less and went in for "sitting" activities. They spent four times as many hours watching TV as the others. Similar studies on boys revealed the same pattern.

A growing number of physicians who specialize in obesity agree with Mayer. They believe that obesity is a physical activity problem; not a nutrition problem. Several years ago, *Lancet*, the highly respected British medical journal, summed it up in one brief sentence: "In obesity, sloth may be more important than gluttony."

Dieting Isn't Enough

That sentence seems to imply that putting an end to gluttony does not produce the desired lean, healthy look. This has been the observation of people who have lost weight. They often complain that they still look flabby. The reason is that when most people diet to lose weight, they lose both fat and lean body tissue. Lean body tissue is the bone-muscle-organ tissue of your body. Lean body tissue gives you your shape, and you don't want to lose it. A loss of lean tissue causes a saggy appearance. Exercise is better than dieting, then, because activity burns up fat but will not cause you to lose lean body tissue.

While at Kent State University, Dr. William Zuti and Dr. Lawrence Golding conducted a study that illustrates this point nicely. They set out to compare the effects of several different methods of weight reduction on the body. The 25 women who participated in the study were all between the ages of 25 and 40 and were 20 to 40 pounds overweight. Three groups were formed: (1) eight women who dieted only, reducing their caloric intake by 500 calories a day but holding their physical activity constant; (2) nine who continued to eat as usual, but increased their physical activity to burn off 500 extra calories a day; and (3) eight who reduced their caloric intake by 250 calories a day and increased physical activity to burn off another 250 calories. Before and after the 16-week period, the subjects were tested for body weight, body density, skin fold and girth measurements, and selected blood fats.

By the end of the study, women in all three groups had lost about the same amount of weight. The average individual weight loss in each group was 11.4 pounds, proof that all the methods were extremely effective in controlling weight. However, the significant finding of the study was that there was a difference in body composition.

Those in the diet-only group lost some fat, but they also lost some lean body tissue; those in the combination diet-exercise group lost more fat than the dieters, and actually gained some lean tissue; the exercise group lost about the same amount of fat as the combination group, but they gained the greatest amount of lean tissue. The women in the exercise group were judged to look best by the end of the program.

The members of the exercise group also had more stamina than the others; their circulatory systems were much better able to withstand the rigors of exercise. The report concluded that the use of exercise in a weight reduction program is far superior to dieting alone in its effect on body composition and physical fitness.

TABLE 1. HOW MUCH EXERCISE IS NECESSARY FOR WEIGHT CONTROL?

It has been estimated that you must walk a minimum of 30 minutes a day, four days a week, at your target heart rate level to make desirable weight and appearance changes. That way the changes will occur in a consistent manner.

Number Of Calories Expended By Walking (Per Hour)							
Walking Speed in mph	Weight in Pounds						
	100	120	140	160	180	200	220
2	130	160	185	210	240	265	290
2½	155	185	220	250	280	310	345
3	180	215	250	285	325	360	395
3½	205	248	290	330	375	415	455
4	235	280	325	375	420	470	515
4½	310	370	435	495	550	620	680
5	385	460	540	615	690	770	845

Walking also helps people to get out of the guilt trap of dieting. People who exercise regularly realize that they can "cheat" a little on special occasions without feeling guilty. They know that if they eat too much, they can simply walk a little extra distance to burn up those extra calories. They have the right idea. They have learned how to pay the price for living in modern-day America. And they like the way they look.

Experimental research provides hundreds of successful cases, but an informal experiment by Golding at Kent State University may be the most convincing one. Golding conducted a vigorous exercise program at the University for 17 years, in which more than 100 men participated on a long-term basis. Each year he took pictures of the men as part of his testing procedure. Since the men had been in the program for such a long period of time, they started to change significantly in fitness. Their appearance also changed. A favorite game of Golding's was to give the year-by-year pictures of one of these men to his graduate students. He would block off the face and head on each picture so no one could see the obvious indications of aging (wrinkles, balding, etc.). He would then ask each student to arrange the man's photographs in a proper chronological order. The students consistently positioned them backward.

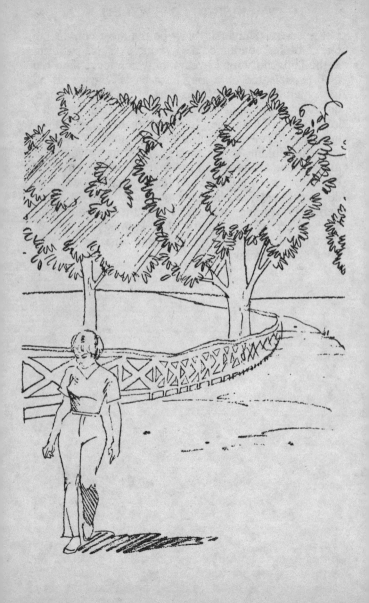

WALKING TO
RELIEVE STRESS

A WALK IS AS GOOD FOR YOUR MIND
AS IT IS FOR YOUR BODY.

Henry Thoreau did it. Harry Truman, Abe Lincoln, and Albert Einstein did it. Robert Louis Stevenson, Adlai Stevenson, Conrad Adenauer, and Paul Dudley White were all members of the walking fraternity. Many famous people extolled the virtues of walking. Their day was incomplete without their "daily constitutional."

They weren't successful because they walked, but walking certainly helped them become more complete beings. They got more out of life. Walking helped relax and recharge their minds and bodies.

Recently, scientists have tried to explain why walking exercises your mind. Dr. Paul Dudley White, dean of American cardiologists, said, "A minimum of an hour a day of fast walking . . . is absolutely necessary for one's optimal health, including that of the brain."

Unfortunately, many people are unaware of the relationship between walking and the mind. To these people, the mind and the body are separate entities. Yet your physical condition affects your psychological well-being and vice versa. This isn't a new idea. The average urban person is underactive but overstimulated. Actual physical danger is rare, but stress and anxiety are prevalent. You are not challenged by saber-toothed tigers or invading barbarians the way your ancestors were. Instead, your boss yells at you, you're pressured to meet deadlines, or you have to rush to catch a plane. You confront many frustrating domestic and social demands. Stress is brought about by money and personal problems, overcrowding, unrelenting noise, anxiety about inflation, fuel shortages, crime, war, and . . . well, you get the picture.

Coping with these kinds of problems requires you to use your head rather than your fists, but your body prepares for "fist" action anyway. The cerebral cortex of the brain sees a threat and signals the hypothalamus, which switches on the nervous and endocrine systems. The nervous system in turn stimulates the liver, which increases the blood's clotting ability (reducing the likelihood of your bleeding to death should you be injured). Fat stored in the body is readied for conversion into energy. The heart rate speeds up to send extra oxygen to the muscles. Muscle tension increases to facilitate quick responses. Large amounts of hormones are released to allow the body to engage in long periods of intense activity. All this happens automatically in response to a threat, whether it's real or imagined.

Today this physical response to threats is outmoded. After all, we're "civilized." In most instances, we hide our natural responses because fighting or running away is inappropriate. We learn to mask anger and bottle up our frustrations and anxieties. The natural, physical response is thwarted, and this causes more tension.

This results in a tremendous energy drain. It can ultimately lead to high blood pressure and dangerous changes in blood chemistry. What can these lead to? You name it: obesity; ulcers; colitis; muscle twitches and tics; high blood pressure; heart disease; cancer; emotional disorders such as neurosis, anxiety, depression, and various compulsions. They're all there, the host of 20th-century maladies we have all come to know and live with—and fear. Each of these ailments, physical and emotional, can cause more tension. The cycle whirls and widens.

So get off the cycle: walk. Walking can release tension, provide an outlet for pent-up emotions, and release hormones and blood fats that would be harmful if contained in the body.

Charles T. Kuntzleman considers himself a good example of what walking can do to relieve stress. "I lead a pretty hectic life," he says. "I have five children, two dogs, serve as a consultant on two programs for the National YMCA, travel constantly, write about two books a year. . . and on and on. I run on 'hype' all the time. Yet I have found a 30- to 45-minute walk extremely relaxing. Before going to bed for the night, my wife and I like to take our walk. It's quiet, a time for us to be together. There are fewer cars on the road. All seems so serene. My day unwinds. Things are put into perspective. After the walk we get ready for bed. And from there on it's a race to see if I can stay awake until my head hits the pillow."

George Trevalyan, the famous historian, said, "I never knew a man to go for an honest day's walk for whatever distance, great or small . . . and not have his reward in the repossession of the soul."

Exercise experts agree that release of nervous tension is one of the most important functions of walking. They've been saying it for years. Recently, Dr. Hans Selye, world-famous endocrinologist, put it this way: "A voluntary change of activity is as good or even better than rest . . . for example, when either fatigue or forced interruption prevents us from finishing a mathematical problem, it is better to go for a swim than simply sit around. . . . Stress on one system helps to relax another."

The effectiveness of walking on reducing tension has been measured in the laboratory. Dr. Herbert deVries, an exercise physiologist at the University of Southern California, examined a group of men 50 years of age and over. All had a history of migraine headaches. He found that after a few weeks of regular physical activity, the headaches disappeared—without medication. (As you may know, the accepted theory about migraines is that they are somehow caused by tension.) In a second study, deVries discovered that a 15-minute walk reduced neuromuscular tension more effectively than did a standard dosage of tranquilizers. DeVries concluded that exercise can be more relaxing than medication.

The question is: How does walking reduce tension? There are several theories. It may just be escape—from big problems like international conflicts as well as smaller hassles such as the telephone, the children, parents, and occupational frustrations. Walking is a mini-vacation—a vacation in the middle of the day, in the evening, or in the morning. It's a vacation that no one can take away from you. You don't have to worry about a thing. Your vacation can be short or quite long. You're free.

Less Anxiety, Lower Blood Pressure

Anxiety is closely related to tension. No one knows exactly how they are related, but doctors know there is a connection. It's like the chicken and the egg: no one knows which came first. A lot of people are in fitness classes because they are too anxious. Their doctors realize that activity can reduce anxiety, so they recommended exercise.

Infrequent anxiety does little harm. But constant anxiety can cause problems. One of those problems is hypertension.

A man we'll call Hal is a good example. He was one of the 22 million Americans with a hypertensive condition of unknown cause. Hal's blood pressure was 180/110 when his doctor suggested exercise as a possible way of reducing it. (Normal is around 140/90 or less.) Hal's doctor said Hal was an extremely anxious individual. An exercise program was prescribed, with the caution that Hal should proceed slowly, very slowly, at first. His blood pressure would be closely watched. His doctor and Charles T. Kuntzleman decided that a daily walk of one to two miles would be sufficient for the first few months. Hal enrolled in a fitness class.

Within a few weeks, Hal's blood pressure dropped to 165–170/100—an encouraging sign. And it continued to decline until, at the end of 18 weeks, it had stabilized at about 155–160/98. At this point Hal left the class and started his own program of vigorous walking and some swimming. His blood pressure continued to drop over the next year and finally stabilized at 140/90, which is high normal. Hal also reported fewer headaches than before (quite possibly the headaches were tied to the hypertensive condition). By the end of the year of regular physical activity, his weight had dropped by 28 pounds and his percent of total body fat went from 31 to 18 percent. Of course this didn't all happen just because of Hal's exercise program. Hal's doctor put him on a diet and limited his use of sugar, salt, and cholesterol. But the doctor felt the most significant factor in his reduced blood pressure was exercise.

Nathalie Smith had high blood pressure too. Her doctor recorded a blood pressure of 200/115. Anxious and tense, she complained of not being able to remember names, dates, and events. The doctor was so upset that he was afraid to let her drive home—he feared she would have a stroke. She was on drug therapy, but she complained that the drugs made her feel "spacy." At first the idea of walking scared her. She felt so poorly she didn't want to walk. She was afraid it would harm her. But she tried it. Half a mile was as much as she could handle. Even then she was exhausted by the time she finished. In fact, while walking the half mile, she had to rest frequently. But she stuck with it. Over three years her fitness level improved. She walked farther and faster. Now, at age 67, she walks four to six miles a day. And the six miles is easy. She refuses to miss a day. Her walk is vitally important to her. When asked why she walks, she says, "I'm afraid if I stop, I'll start to feel lousy again. I feel so good now I just don't want to stop."

Some other symptoms of anxiety have disappeared. She had often been certain she was going to have a heart attack: she used to wake up at night, her heart pounding and fluttering. But since she started walking, that problem has disappeared. Leg cramps that used to bother her at night are also gone.

Today, Nathalie Smith is a new person. She enjoys her good health. She gets more out of life than she did three, four, five, or even six years ago. She no longer feels the anxiety and tension she once did. And her blood pressure is now 118/78.

These cases aren't flukes. Exercise alone has often proved successful in lowering and stabilizing dynamic blood pressure. It even seems to affect resting blood pressure. Dr. Jack Rudd, of Boston's Veteran Administration Outpatient Clinic, and William Day, Ph.D., former physical director of the Cambridge, Massachusetts, YMCA, put 19 middle-aged and elderly hypertensive men on an exercise program incorporating brisk walking, calisthenics, running, cycling, and swimming. Before the program, the average level of blood pressure for the men was 155/95; after six weeks it was down to 133/85.

Walking or exercise alone will not alleviate all cases of hypertension. But one thing is clear: it often does produce excellent results. (It works best for people who are overly anxious.) However, no one ought to begin an exercise program on a do-it-yourself basis to relieve a hypertensive condition. Anyone with high blood pressure should get medical clearance before engaging in increased physical activity—even walking.

Psychologists and psychiatrists have made exercise part of anxiety therapy. Some very interesting work done by Dr. Richard Driscoll shows how it works. Driscoll, a psychologist at Eastern State Psychiatric Hospital in Knoxville, Tennessee, asked people to exercise and to think pleasant thoughts. (Most walkers say they can't help but have pleasant thoughts while walking.)

Driscoll's report states that his prescription substantially reduced anxiety. He has some theories about why physical activity helps reduce anxiety. He says that activity and anxiety both trigger responses in the sympathetic nervous system that prepare the body for vigorous activity. This has long been known as the body's response to danger. These physical changes are also known to be the body's way of preparing for exercise. When the heightened physical state is a prelude to exercise, we make use of the tension and stimulation. When you feel that way because you are anxious, exercise can provide a vent for your anxiety.

Driscoll offers two additional explanations of why exercise helps lower anxiety. First, physical exertion is intentional. It requires attention, effort, and motivation. It usually inspires a feeling of commitment and accomplishment. These constructive feelings probably relieve anxiety by making use of some of the bottled-up tension. Second, for many persons, physical exertion is associated with excitement, assertiveness, and friendship. These positive feelings may also help to relieve anxious feelings.

The standard medical concept, "Action absorbs anxiety," says it all.

Relief from Depression

Exercise also seems to help short-circuit depression. The term depression is a catch-all which may include everything from the blahs to psychosis. Depression is a serious problem in our society. Doctors tell us that over 10 percent of the population will score in the "depressed" range on what is known as a depression questionnaire. Some hospitals are reporting that over half the patients coming to their clinics list depression as their primary problem.

Doctors are now excited by reports that seem to show that exercise, such as walking, can relieve a person's depression. Although most of the studies to date have been done on running, we believe the conclusions can be extended to walking as well. Anything that is repetitive in nature, that allows people to relax, and gives them a feeling of accomplishment seems to be helpful in reducing depression. Here are several reasons why.

1. Walking regularly requires patience. A person learns through walking that it takes time to make significant physical changes. An appreciation of the value of patience may reduce depression.
2. Walkers learn, often dramatically, that they can change themselves for the better. They see that they are sufficiently in control of their lives to be able to improve their health, appearance and self-image.
3. In this way they develop a feeling of accomplishment. Any time you experience a sense of success, you will probably be pulled out of depression.

There's an old comedy routine about a doctor who steps on his patient's foot to make the patient forget about his headache. There's something of that in the relationship between walking and depression. Walkers are forced to notice new and significant body sensations, which distract them. People who walk tend to focus on their sore calves or other muscle groups and forget about the annoying physical symptoms of depression.

These changes can make walking almost addictive. Many people find they need their walk as much as others need their morning cup of coffee. According to Dr. William Glasser, physician and author of *Positive Addiction,* walkers transform a negative addiction into a positive one. They start to give up such things as smoking, drinking, overeating, and nonproductive arguing.

The National Institute on Mental Health is currently investigating the biochemical changes that occur in the brain when a person exercises. Depressed people placed on a regular exercise program apparently have mood elevations.

Naturalist Donald Culross Peattie said: "I've often started off on a walk in the state called mad—mad in the sense of sore-headed, or mad with tedium or confusion; I've set forth dull, null, and even thoroughly discouraged. But I never came back in such a frame of mind, and I have never met a human being whose humor was not the better for a walk."

Walking to Euphoria

If you talk to long-distance runners, they'll tell you about the euphoria they experience after running 30 or 40 minutes. It's called a "runner's high." Many people who have participated in walking programs have experienced the same kind of thing by seeing their world at three to four and a half miles an hour. They feel a period of heightened consciousness; they feel more creative, enthusiastic, excited. Some psychologists feel that this "high" is an altered state of consciousness, an opening up of the unconscious.

Thought processes are altered. Problems seem to become less important and many are let go. It's almost as if there were a psychiatrist inside of you, solving your problems as you walk.

Dr. Arthur Kovacs, a Los Angeles clinical psychologist, uses long-distance walking as part of the therapy for his patients. He says, "the experience of being out in the wilderness adds another dimension to the psychotherapy experience. . . . It allows an individual to relate to his body. It also allows him to improve his self-concept by showing himself competent in an area."

Some experts have tried to show that exercise and walking improve circulation; that this improved circulation sends the brain more oxygen, which brings on the euphoria.

(An experimental study done by clinical psychologists at the Veteran's Administration Hospital in Buffalo, New York, supported this "greater oxygen to the brain" thesis. Pure oxygen was administered to senile patients placed in a pressurized chamber. As a result, the patients' mental alertness improved. After being treated with oxygen twice a day for 15 days, these elderly people took a standard memory test and scored as much as 25 percent better than they had before the oxygen therapy.)

Increased Productivity, Creativity

Kuntzleman, fitness advisor to CONSUMER GUIDE® and contributing editor of this book, says he is convinced that a walking program can improve a person's productivity.

Several years ago I offered a fitness class to the employees of a middle-sized corporation. The class consisted of 10 minutes of aerobic exercise, twice daily, every working day. Thirty women participated. The aerobic exercise was divided into group sessions in which people could exercise to music or take a walk. These people were dedicated: they came to three to four sessions a week.

After two years, I noticed the typical physical changes in the participants: loss of weight, better appearance, and trimmer bodies. But the most striking changes were psychological. The participants kept telling me: "I feel better, happier, and more productive." I was intrigued. I had seen some of the changes that take place in people when they become more active. I'd even experienced many of them myself. But I'd never been in the position to watch this phenomenon take place step by step. And here it was happening right before my eyes.

At this point, I decided to keep track of what was happening. I wanted to find out what was really going on. The statements that some of the women made about having more energy and being able to get more work done were especially interesting. Was it just a feeling, or was there really something to it?

I didn't have a budget to hire a psychologist, and I didn't feel qualified to administer psychological tests. But I decided that one good way to measure the women's changed attitudes would be to check the personnel records of the women in the exercise program. I found they missed an average of 2.37 work days during the first year of the program. I then selected a control group of 30 nonexercising women and checked their attendance records. They missed an average of 4.28 days.

It was possible, of course, that the exercise group was more highly motivated to begin with. To check on this, I compared the two groups' attendance records before the exercise class began. Prior to the class, the women who would become the exercises had missed an average of 3.43 work days; others had missed 3.3 days. This convinced me that productivity can be improved with proper exercise.

Often our busy schedules prevent us from doing the kind of reflection that seems necessary to the creative process. We get wrapped up in our daily routines and do things out of habit. We feel we should spend more time alone—thinking, perhaps meditating—but we are filled with so much nervous energy we can't sit still. The calm solitude of walking outdoors gives you a chance to work things out in your mind. New ideas to help you solve old problems are likely to pop into your head while you walk. This does not seem likely to occur while you watch TV or worry. Former Supreme Court Justice William O. Douglas said that when he had a knotty legal case to consider, the best thing he could do was to go for a walk. The answer would come to him in a flash.

Dr. George Sheehan has said, "Never trust an idea lying down." Here's our advice: When you can't solve a problem, go for a walk.

SLOWING DOWN
THE AGING PROCESS

WALKING CAN ADD YEARS TO YOUR LIFE, AND LIFE TO YOUR YEARS.

We're about to tell you a very sad story—sad but true. It's an American tragedy.

A woman we'll call Sally is respected and loved by her family and her friends; yet she's not happy. Her age is 58, but if you saw her, you'd think her closer to 85. Completely sedentary since childhood, she is near the bottom on the physical fitness scale. She can't keep up with her husband or her children. Instead, she spends most all of her time in her house, waiting for a heart attack. She has many excuses for staying indoors: it's too hot outside, too cold, too windy. Sally is miserable, and old before her time.

Middle age, it has been said, is the time when the narrow waistline and the broad mind change places. That's clever, but not very amusing when we think of people like Sally. There's no way that any of us can avoid growing old. But we can do something to assure that we'll age gracefully and continue to enjoy life to the fullest every day.

Dr. Ernst Jokl of the University of Kentucky has said, "There is little doubt that proper physical activity as part of a way of life can significantly delay the aging process." The editors of this book are convinced that a walking program such as the one we'll introduce to you shortly can add years to your life and life to your years.

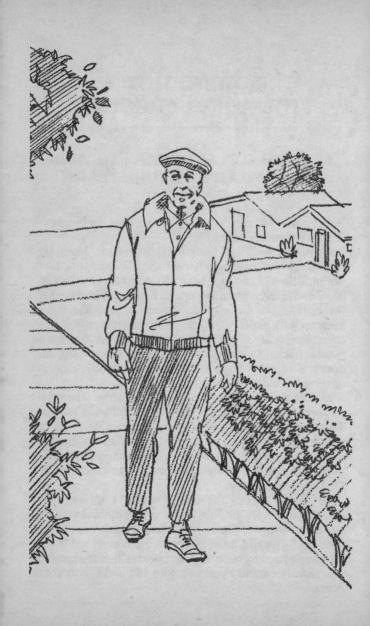

Many changes occur as we get older. Among the most common are fatigue, decreased vigor and strength, increased weight, reduced joint flexibility, a change in bowel and bladder habits, a decline in sex drive, failing sight and hearing, a decrease in mental agility, and general lack of stamina.

The process of aging varies a great deal from one person to another. It's impossible to determine the exact time of life when it will begin. We usually associate aging with the age of 65 or so, but the signs begin to appear in most of us as early as 30 or 35 years of age. Some people seem washed out before the age of 40. On the other hand, we all know people who seem young and vigorous at 60 or 70 years of age.

Although the average American probably assumes that the changes that occur after the age of 30 are a natural part of the aging process, this is probably incorrect. Current research suggests that such change may be the result not of passing years, but a passive life style. For example, Dr. Bengt Saltin and his associates in Sweden placed five healthy young men in bed for 20 days. After the bed rest, Saltin found that the maximum cardiac output of the men decreased 26 percent, their maximum oxygen uptake dropped 27 percent, and their exercise stroke volume and maximum breathing capacity fell 30 percent. Even their amount of lean body tissue decreased.

Dr. Matti J. Karvonen of Finland describes the most interesting aspect of the relationship between exercise and aging. The phenomena of aging are the reverse of those caused by exercise training. In some populations, a decrease in the amount of habitual exercise accentuates several "age" changes; in others with lifelong exercise, the state of training delays them. Karvonen says long-term exercise may have a positive effect on health, even if it does not prolong life. Such an effect would be manifested by a lower frequency of illness throughout one's life.

The later years of life—particularly those of retirement—should be happy, dynamic years. The retirement years can be truly rewarding, if you have energy and vitality. But the promise of a full life in our later years comes only to those who are healthy, alert, robust, and active. Unfortunately for too many Americans, the dream of a happy, healthy retirement never comes true.

Most people make financial plans for their retirement. They have financial resources they hope will ensure happiness. However, many have neglected their physical resources. By the time they are 60, their stamina has faltered, their weight has escalated, and their general health has declined. Suddenly, their financial resources are no longer as important as they once were. The concern for wealth gives way to concern for health.

Fortunately, regardless of your age, you can do something about your health that will start producing dividends and returns almost immediately. Even if you have let your physical well-being slip because of social, financial, and family demands, you can make improvements. You can become more active and improve your level of physical performance so you'll enjoy life more. But you can't just wish for it. You must take an active role in slowing down the aging process, and you must start now.

New Meaning for "Life Insurance"

The American Heart Association says, "Walking briskly, not just strolling, is the simplest and also one of the best forms of exercise." The Metropolitan Life Insurance Company says: "Exercise does not have to be either laborious or time consuming. One of the simplest ways is to walk when you do not absolutely have to ride. Walking is a fine way to keep yourself in good shape." Those statements should impress you. After all, insurance companies want you to stay alive.

Dr. Harry J. Johnson, former medical director for the Life Extension Institute, said it well. Walking, he said, "will not keep you young, mind you; inevitably the body changes with time. But it can keep you middle-aged for life. It lengthens the middle-age plateau and keeps you from getting old before your time." Middle-aged for life: perhaps it's not the mythical fountain of youth, but it's the next best thing.

Walking is safe for people in their later years. It can be tailor-made to individual differences and fitness levels.

Before we go any further, we want to ask a favor: please read this book all the way through—or at least to the end of the next chapter—before you begin a walking program of your own. No matter what your age, and especially if you are approaching or are beyond middle age, you'll want to read what we have to say about asking your doctor's advice. We've spent a great deal of time trying to inspire you to get yourself into shape. We want you to be inspired; we also want you to be careful.

Dr. Theodore Klumpp, an avid 75-year-old walker, says:

Fundamentally, the value of walking for older people in keeping fit depends upon two things. First, the condition of the person and second, how he goes about walking. Regarding his physical condition: if he walks at a brisk pace and stays within his capabilities, walking is a very good exercise for older people. Regarding his method of walking: mild stress is necessary to keep the cardiovascular system in good condition. We've built into our system a pretty good barometer to tell us how much or how little exercise we should take. This barometer is your feelings of fatigue, breathlessness, and the development of other unpleasant symptoms. When walking, even if older, you must increase your pulse rate and press to the point of slight breathlessness. That way you'll condition your cardiovascular condition and improve the tone of your cardiovascular system.

You don't have to be afraid to walk just because you're getting older. You might have slowed down a bit and lost a little flexibility over the years, but that doesn't mean you have to live like poor old Sally. All you have to do is take it easy at the start and listen to your body.

If Eula Weaver can do it, you surely can. At age 77, Ms. Weaver suffered her first heart attack. It was a severe one. She was placed on several types of medication and was told to go home and wait for the inevitable—a fatal heart attack. Another physician who examined her said, "Eula, you can do that or you can do something about your condition. You'll feel a lot better if you start to walk." Walking seemed impossible to her: she had a difficult time getting to the front door. But she decided to give it a try. Each day she tried to walk a little bit more than the day before. Soon she was walking a mile a day. Her mental attitude improved. Her physical condition dramatically changed. Today, at 89, Eula continues to walk regularly. She also jogs—she even holds her age group record for the 880-yard run. That's not bad for a woman who was told 12 years ago to go home and wait.

Orville Fitzgerald shows that Eula Weaver's success was no fluke. Fitzgerald was a barber for 45 years. One spring morning, at the age of 66, he suffered a severe heart attack. He was hospitalized and later told to slow down. He closed his barber shop. People cautioned him not to exercise. Fitzgerald didn't listen to them; he took his doctor's advice instead. He started walking. At first a block was plenty. But each day he would try to go a little farther. He took his nitroglycerin along to help reduce any chest pain or heart palpitations. Some people were concerned about him, but that didn't slow him down. He says he was afraid to stop. "Too many people who just sit end up back in the hospital," he told us. After a few months, he was walking three miles a day. He felt terrific. His post-attack depression disappeared. His legs became stronger. His wind grew better. And his quality of life improved dramatically. He says, "Walking is basic for my recovery mentality. It has made me optimistic. I can see life again and God's green earth. Walking brought me back. I would exhort anyone who has had a heart attack to walk for recovery."

That was three years ago. Today, Fitzgerald is barbering again, only this time it's at his local community care center. He is scheduled for four hours a day and usually puts in four to six. Sometimes he puts in eight.

The point of these stories is obvious. The human body is tough. It can withstand a lot of physical strain. Most people don't give their bodies enough credit. Dr. Paul Dudley White often said physicians just don't realize how tough the body is. He would then point with pride to President Dwight D. Eisenhower, who had suffered several heart attacks yet lived a full, vigorous life. White said anyone else would have died as a result of such damage; but not Eisenhower. The President relied on his body's toughness. With the help of some good preventive measures given to him by White, Eisenhower was able to bounce back.

Martha's story is another example of how resilient the human body can be. At the age of 77, Martha had her first coronary. During the next few years, she suffered at least two more heart attacks and had some very serious chest pains, heart irregularities, and tremendous fatigue. Her symptoms were diagnosed as heart failure. After years of faithful service, her heart was giving out. The doctor gave her various kinds of medication and specific instructions not to exercise. Martha turned in on herself. She did less and less. After a period of time she wouldn't get out of bed by herself, but relied on her daughter to help her. She refused to dress herself. She wouldn't prepare meals. Her condition deteriorated.

A woman who lived next door—an avid walker—went over and talked to Martha one day. The woman said, "Martha, you can sit here and fear the grim reaper or you can do something about your life. How about going for a walk with me?" Martha was startled, but she listened. At first Martha and her friend walked to the front door, then gradually to the mailbox. Slowly the distances increased. After a period of about six months, they walked about three-quarters of a mile.

Some interesting changes occurred. Martha began to dress herself and prepare her own meals; she took the wash off her clothesline without help; she went to church; and she began to look forward to her walks.

Can't Walking Be Harmful?

Since 1967 almost 1,000 people (85 percent of whom had diagnosed heart disease) have participated in the Cardiac Pulmonary Resuscitation Institute (CAPRI) Program of Seattle, Washington. Patients in the program walk fast or jog one hour a day, three times a week. In nine years there have been 15 incidents of patient collapse during exercise. (All were successfully resuscitated.) At first that may sound excessive. But the patients had logged over 116,000 hours of activity. That means that there was one collapse every 7,700 hours. Certainly, one collapse is still a serious matter. But those are still pretty good odds, and they look even better when you consider what the odds of the patients would have been had they not engaged in the program. Most of those people were headed for deadly heart attacks.

Further surveys on cardiac rehabilitation programs are even more impressive. Dr. William Haskell of

Stanford University reporting at the American Heart Association meeting in 1975 stated that you can expect one collapse every 17,585 hours and one fatal collapse every 94,957 hours. This means the risk of death for cardiac patients while exercising in a medically supervised exercise program is about the same as that reported for cardiac patients in general.

Research has shown that older people can withstand great amounts of exercise. In fact, since most of them were very active during their childhood and young adult years (there were few automobiles or school buses back then), they have a good base. And they are able to pick up exercise quite well. Many, once conditioned, seem to have more stamina than the average teenager of today.

Recent Research on Aging

In recent years there has been an increase in research on the problems of aging. The studies state that the control of senescence—the fight against aging—should begin as early as possible, and exercise is an excellent way to do it. The heart, brain, regulatory functions, and the whole body benefit.

How much difference exercise can make is shown in studies of long-lived Russian peasants. David Kaliashvili, a cardiologist, found that many of these older people had forms of heart and blood vessel diseases, but the oxygen supply to their hearts was so good as a result of collateral circulation that heart attacks went unnoticed and did little harm. The collateral circulation (additional circulation caused by the opening of new blood vessels), Kaliashvili said, was the result of an active life style. In other words, exercise didn't hurt them. And it won't harm you. You can walk without fear, provided you follow the principles outlined in this book.

A three-day conference on exercise and aging held at the National Institute of Health in Bethesda, Maryland, spelled out the relationship between exercise and aging.

1. Walking is the most efficient form of exercise—and the only one you can safely follow all the years of your life.

2. As people get older, their bones start to demineralize and lose their resistance to breaking. Exercise, such as walking, slows the bone demineralization process, particularly in the legs. Through exercise your bone-growing cells are stimulated. Bones remain tougher and less likely to break. This also promotes a greater range of motion.

   (A Reno, Nevada, orthopedic clinic did extensive tests on a man, at least 60 years old, who has exercised vigorously for the past 12 years. The tests included x-rays of his legs. At the conclusion of their study, one of the doctors sent a letter to him which said, "Your bone age is approximately 12 years less than your chronological age. This indicates to me that your exercising has been effective in slowing the aging process.")

3. As people get older, particularly those who have smoked or who have worked in high-pollution areas, they develop emphysema-like changes in their lungs. Those individuals who exercise may still exhibit such changes, but they still have far greater capacity than sedentary people.

4. As you age, your cardiovascular function declines. It loses its elasticity and vigorousness. Yet the cardiovascular systems of older Americans who exercise show a maximum preservation of function.

5. One obvious phenomenon of aging is an increase in obesity. As people get into their 40s, 50s, and 60s, their weight escalates. So does their percentage of body fat. This condition greatly affects health. But exercise is a strong deterrent to obesity.

6. Closely related to obesity is the fact that as people get older they tend to eat less than they used to in an effort to keep their weight under control. When they do this, their nutrition often suffers. Daily exercise permits greater food intake and better blood circulation, which improves each cell's nourishment while preventing obesity.

7. Besides heart disease and cancer, many older Americans fear late-onset diabetes. Even though this disease can be controlled, it kills, maims, and reduces a person's well-being. Interestingly, late-onset diabetes is almost entirely reversible by exercise if you are overweight.

8. Rheumatoid arthritis and osteoarthritis are common in older people. It has been estimated that over 90 percent of all Americans over the ago of 60 have some form of osteoarthritis. The conference studies showed that arthritics can perhaps benefit the most of all older people from exercise—provided the exercise is increased slowly but steadily.

9. Many Americans fear getting older. They fear that they will be "turned out to pasture," become unwanted. This increases stress, depression, and fear. Walking seems to stem the tide. Exercise improves the quality of life. Research comparing exercise to a widely prescribed tranquilizer found exercise to be superior in relaxing and elevating one's mood—with none of the drug's side-effects.

In other words, experts and researchers on aging today see the wisdom in the statement that "walking is man's best medicine." That statement came from Hippocrates, the father of medicine, over 2,000 years ago.

Many older Americans today claim they are regimented, merely tolerated by society rather than being considered vital and valued members of it. One excellent way to escape that regimentation is by taking part in what we call the fitness revolution. Choose to walk while everyone else is riding. Go for a nice vigorous walk when everyone else is cemented to an easy chair. Condition your body while others let theirs go to pot. When you get into the real spirit of the revolution, you can always dream up your own personal ways of showing your physical individuality. And you'll find that you've never had more fun.

If you're going to break out of your sedentary rut for good, you will have to get rid of the excuses for not exercising. But, of course, it must be done carefully and thoughtfully. Enthusiasm should be directed to the goal of moving closer to fitness every day, not to setting records. Don't let your enthusiasm trick you into overdoing it. Starting a walking program with a 10-mile hike is foolish. Do most exercises gently, being careful not to put too much stress on your legs and ankles.

Inserting a new activity into your life means that you may have to leave something else out. You need to take stock of your priorities. When you stop to think about it, how many things are more important than your health and well-being?

A few years ago a man we know found an interesting solution to what could be a problem for many older walkers. He began walking to and from work every day, a distance of several miles. Much of the route took him along a narrow country road. In late autumn, the early sunset made it necessary for him to walk home in the dark, which made his wife nervous. On the verge of giving up his walking, he did some thinking and realized he could walk to work in the morning, then walk home at noon and get his car. A fitness problem was licked in a simple and obvious way.

The old saying, "It's never too late" certainly applies to walking. It is one of the best ways to break out of the sedentary rut. Just start your mind working in the right direction; your legs will follow right along.

If you begin exercising as we've suggested, will you live to be 100? Probably not; yet you have a better chance of reaching that age if you do exercise than you have if you don't. Exercise will put you in better physical condition. It can slow the aging process— sometimes by many years. And it makes you feel younger. With these benefits, how can you lose?

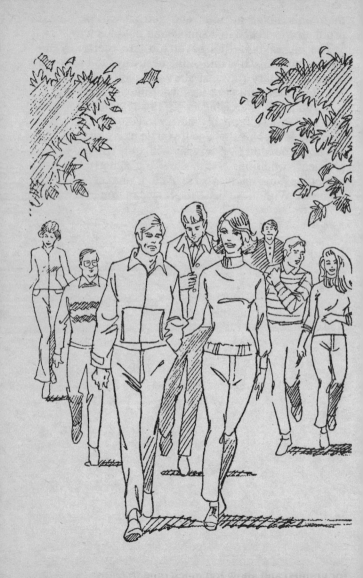

THE CONSUMER GUIDE®
WALKING PROGRAM

OUR PROVEN METHOD ENABLES YOU
TO GET THE MOST FROM
EVERY WALK.

You acquired your walking skills when you were between the ages of nine months and two years, so you don't need us or anyone else to tell you how to walk. Although this chapter will lay out some specific instructions that we believe you ought to follow in order to maximize the benefits of a walking program, the "secret" of walking comfortably is to walk naturally—pretty much as you've been walking up to now.

Yet the program we've developed for you amounts to more than a leisurely stroll. To continue to enjoy the rewards of this program, you may eventually find yourself walking for more than an hour, several days a week. Our program allows you to start slowly and progress without strain. However, because we know that some of you will be impatient and will be tempted to push yourselves to hard, we'd like you to answer this question before you go any further: Do you have any questions about your health?

If you do, check with your doctor before you start your walking program. Of course, if you have arthritis, anemia, low back pain, uncontrolled diabetes, or serious diseases of the lungs, kidneys, liver or heart, you ought to be seeing a doctor regularly anyway. But many Americans have a tendency to take their health for granted and allow too much time to elapse between physical examinations. Those of you who have questions about your health should get a check-up. That check-up should include an examination of your heart, blood vessels, muscles, and joints. Ideally your blood would be analyzed for cholesterol and triglycerides, and your blood pressure would be noted. A resting electrocardiogram (ECG) should also be performed.

In some cases, it may be a good idea to take an exercise stress test, which is nothing more than an electrocardiogram that is taken while you are exercising.

Dr. Kenneth Cooper's recommendations in the *Journal of the American Medical Association* are good ones. According to Cooper:

> If you are under 30, you can start exercising if you've had a check-up in the past year and your doctor found nothing wrong with you; if you are between 30 and 39, you should have a check-up within three months before you start exercising, and the examination should include an electrocardiogram (ECG) taken at rest; if you are between 40 and 59, your guidelines are the same as those for the 30–39 group, plus an ECG taken while you are exercising; if you are over 59, you should follow the same requirements as for the 40–59 group, and the examination should be performed immediately before you embark on any exercise program.

But an examination (with or without a stress test) isn't the final answer. Let's face it, not all doctors understand exercise. Some have negative attitudes about it. So here is some further advice. Before following your doctor's advice on exercise, check these things out:

1. Look at your physician's waistline. If it seems too big, don't trust his exercise advice.

2. Make sure your doctor is a nonsmoker.
3. Find out if he is taking part in an aerobic exercise program; that is, exercising three or more times a week. (Golf does not qualify.)

If he passes these three hurdles, then tell him you are going to participate in a walking program. Show him this book, referring to this chapter. Then ask the following:

1. Can you clear me for participation in this program?
2. How long, how hard, and how often am I permitted to exercise?

If your doctor realizes you're serious about exercising, he or she should be pleased. But if he or she reacts with a comment like "Remember, if you walk one mile from home you'll have to walk one mile back," get a second opinion from another doctor.

Doctors deal with sickness, not well-being, so they tend to think in negative rather than positive terms. Don't forget, it's your health. You want to make sure what you're doing is right. You want to obtain the best advice possible.

After your doctor has given you the go-ahead, you may become concerned about proper walking style. Here is *Consumer Guide*® magazine's advice: walk naturally. Your body is unique. It has it's own particular construction and balance, so you can't force it to behave exactly like someone else's.

It is good to keep your spine straight and hold your head high as you walk, but try not to be so conscious of this that you feel unnatural. Don't exaggerate your arm motion. Allow your arms to hang loosely at your sides. They will swing in the opposite action of your legs. Keep your hands, hips, knees and ankles relaxed. As you walk, don't worry about the length of your stride. Just do whatever is comfortable. Each foot should strike the ground at your heel. The weight is then transferred from your heel up along the outer border of your foot toward your toes. Then you should push off with your toes to complete the foot strike pattern. As you move from heel to toe, you will get a rolling motion. Avoid landing flat-footed and on the balls of your feet. If you do, you may be headed for some leg and foot problems later on.

When walking, breathe naturally. If you feel comfortable with your mouth closed, close it. If it seems better open, then open it. Remember, the faster you go the more air you'll need. Help yourself to all the air you want.

Don't follow these guidelines slavishly. It's likely that the way you walk already is best for you. Remember, you're not in a beauty contest. You're walking for fitness and fun. There's no need to worry about style or form.

Three More Important Principles

There are three other principles you ought to follow as you walk.

First, you should be able to hold a conversation with someone beside you as you go. Even when you walk alone, you can use your imagination: do you feel like talking? If not, you can probably conclude that you're walking too fast for your present age or fitness level. This is called the talk test. The talk test is especially important during the first six to 12 weeks of walking.

Second, your walk should be painless. If you experience any chest, jaw, or neck pain, you should slow down. If that doesn't stop the pain, see your doctor and describe what happened. Try to recall the circumstances: "I was walking on a hill," "It occurred during the first few minutes," or "The weather was cold."

Third, if after walking you seem excessively tired

for an hour or longer, the walk was too strenuous. Next time, walk slower and not as far. Your walk should be exhilarating, not fatiguing. If you experience a dizzy or lightheaded feeling, or if your heart is beating too fast while you walk, it's time to back off. If you have a strange hollow feeling in your chest, feel like vomiting, or are tired for at least a day after walking, take it easy. If you can't sleep at night or if your nerves seem shot, it means that you've been pushing too hard. The same is true if you seem to have lost your zing or can't get your breath after a few minutes of exercise. These are your body's warning signs.

All three points emphasize "listening to your body." This listening is something you'll have to learn. But you'll probably find it fun. You'll enjoy your body more. It will let you know when to slow down and when to speed up. You are the best judge of your exercise.

As we have said before, the health of your heart and lungs are critical to your overall well-being. The cells in your body need oxygen to live and grow. Without enough of it, they die. Your lungs take in oxygen and give it to the blood. Your heart pumps blood and the oxygen it is carrying to the cells in your body. The cells take the oxygen from the blood and "burn" it as fuel to grow and work. Anytime something is burned, carbon dioxide is produced. The blood removes this carbon dioxide from your cells; your lungs then send it out into the air.

This process goes on all the time. If your lungs and heart are working properly, you look and feel great. But if your lungs can't take in enough oxygen or if your heart can't pump blood fast enough, your cells can be crippled or killed. This is why any worthwhile physical fitness program must focus on the heart and lungs and how they work together. According to the American Heart Association's Committee on Exercise and Fitness, and the American College of Sports Medicine, an exercise contributes to heart and lung fitness only if it continuously involves both systems for at least 15 minutes or, preferably, 20 minutes or more. That is why a game of tennis, even a very active one, is not the most useful exercise to strengthen the heart and lungs. There may be periods of furious activity, full of lunging and running and rapid stops and starts. But they are too short, and there is too much rest in between. The action is not sustained. Walking, on the other hand, is sustained. It is rhythmical and continuous. This is why it also burns a significant number of calories thus helping to control weight and reduce body fat.

The CONSUMER GUIDE® Walking Program is based on the principle of sustained action. The amount of time spent walking (the amount of sustained action), not the distance or pace, is the crucial part of the program.

Most people measure exercise in terms of time, distance, physical load, or number of actions. Few people think about effort. Effort and work don't mean the same thing. Two people may walk a mile in 15 minutes. Both walk the same distance. But for one person the walk may be effortless, while the other one finds that it is all he can handle. You may be like that second person. If you walk consistently, however, soon walking a mile in 15 minutes won't be difficult at all. Your body will have become more efficient, so you will need less effort to walk the same distance.

So how can you know how much exercise is right? For that matter, how can a program tell you? Your body is not like anyone else's, and it changes from day to day. According to many experts, a computer would be needed to figure out how much activity a particular person needs to benefit from the training effect. Most experts believe that you have a computer built into your body. It's your heart. By exercising at a specific heart rate, you maintain a consistent level of effort. Since your heart reacts to your general condition on a particular day, it will reflect your fatigue, body temperature, and other conditions when you exercise.

Using Your Heart Rate as a Guide

Everyone has what is called a "maximum heart rate." Your maximum heart rate is the number of beats your heart makes per minute when you are running as far, as fast, and as long as possible. (Another term for this is maximum aerobic power level.) Although it varies from person to person, your maximum heart rate is roughly 220 minus your age. If you are 20 years old, your maximum heart rate is about 200; if you are 40, it is about 180.

There is no need for you to exercise at your maximum heart rate level. This could even be dangerous. Fortunately, physiologists have figured out a safe heart range for most people. They call this your target heart rate. Your target heart rate, as it is called in cardiovascular exercise programs, is considered about 70 to 85 percent of your maximum heart rate. That is your optimum level for exercise. That doesn't mean that you can't improve your fitness if your heart rate is above or below this range. It's just that the 70 to 85 percent range is the safest, most efficient range.

Table 1 shows the maximum heart rate, target heart rate range, and the target heart rate for ages 20 to 70 in five-year increments. You may calculate your own rate and range for this chart if your age falls between the ages listed. To use the chart, you must be able to take your pulse. This is very easy.

There are three ways to take your pulse: at the radial artery on your wrist, the temporal artery on your forehead, and the carotid artery on your neck. To take your pulse at your wrist, use the second, third, and fourth fingers of your hand to feel for the pulse along

TABLE 1. YOUR TARGET HEART RATE AND HEART RATE RANGE

Maintaining your target rate is the key to the CONSUMER GUIDE® Walking Program. Your maximum heart rate is the greatest number of beats per minute that your heart is capable of. During exercise, your heart rate should be approximately 75 percent of this maximum. To obtain the cardiovascular benefits of walking—or of any other exercise—maintain a heart rate between 70 percent and 85 percent of your maximum for at least 15, or preferably, 20 minutes. If you exceed 85 percent of your maximum, you are overdoing it and should relax your pace.

Age	Your Maximum Heart Rate (Beats per minute)	Your Target Heart Rate (75 percent of the Maximum in beats per minute)	Your Target Heart Rate Range (Between 70 percent and 85 percent of the Maximum in beats per minute)
20	200	150	140 to 170
25	195	146	137 to 166
30	190	142	133 to 162
35	185	139	130 to 157
40	180	135	126 to 153
45	175	131	123 to 149
50	170	127	119 to 145
55	165	124	116 to 140
60	160	120	112 to 136
65	155	116	109 to 132
70	150	112	105 to 128

the thumb side of your wrist. When you find your pulse (a thump or push), count it for 10 seconds by doing the following. Right before you actually start counting, count the beats by going zero, zero, zero. As soon as the second hand on your watch reaches 12, start counting. First count zero, then one, two, three, four, etc. Stop counting when the second hand reaches the two (10 seconds). Multiply the number you counted by six. The number you get is your pulse. (You can also take your pulse for six seconds and add a zero. This is the easiest and most convenient way, but it can be less accurate.) If you want to take your pulse at your forehead, simply place your third and fourth fingers on your forehead and press. The counting is the same as for the wrist pulse. If you find you can't find your pulse at your wrist or at the forehead, you may use the neck pulse. But if you do this, be careful. Physicians and exercise physiologists frown upon taking a pulse this way. When people place their fingers at their neck, they may develop heart arrhythmias (irregular heart beats). Their pulse rates also may slow down and give a false reading. So if you take your pulse this way, be sure to press lightly.

You now know your target heart rate range and how to take your heart rate. The next step is learning how to keep your heart rate in the proper range when walking. The only way you can do this is by going out and walking. At first you will have to experiment a little, but after a while you will be able to tell whether you are within the range simply by the way you feel.

If you tire quickly and noticeably when you walk within your target heart rate range, reassess your range and lower it. Slow down until you are still working hard but not overexerting yourself. If, on the other hand, you do not feel the effect of your walking, you may have to walk at a faster rate.

A word of caution: Don't be a slave to your pulse rate. Remember the three principles outlined at the beginning of this chapter.

Your maximum heart rate (or maximum aerobic power level) is a difficult measurement to obtain. It requires a great deal of sophisticated equipment, a medical doctor or exercise physiologist, and healthy chunks of time and money. But an accurate reading of your own pulse will give you a good approximation of your maximum aerobic power. Since you can find it without much trouble, you have an easy, inexpensive tool for measuring how strenuously you are exercising.

How to Get Started

Doctors know that most sedentary people develop orthopedic problems by trying to do too much too soon. Dr. Kenneth Cooper, the doctor who made exercise respectable to the medical profession, also found that most people who have had heart attacks while exercising had them within the first few weeks. The problem seems to be an effort to do too much too soon. Some doctors say you should spend at least one month reconditioning yourself for every year you have been sedentary. That's excellent advice.

You need a plan that puts you on a regular walking schedule. We're now going to take you step-by-step through a program that works. It has been tested and perfected over the past five years and has been used by thousands of people all over the United States and Canada. It will make you fit and help you enjoy the true pleasures of walking. You'll find this program demanding enough to get the job done, yet flexible enough to be adapted to your particular needs, age, present level of fitness, and life style.

Don't let the idea of an exercise program scare you off. We won't ask you to do more than you can reasonably do. We just want you to get started, and to keep at it. We want to help you experience the physical, mental, spiritual exhilaration of walking. All the benefits we have described are waiting for you.

The next two tables summarize two starter programs: Starter Program A and Starter Program B. Starter Program A is the one we'd like you to follow. Using this program, you walk at a pace that does not elicit a target heart rate. All you do is walk comfortably and pain-free. Your goal at this point is to get your body ready for more demanding exercise.

TABLE 2. STARTER PROGRAM A

Level 1: Walk 20 minutes a day 4 times a week, or 15 minutes a day 6 times a week.

Level 2: Walk 25 minutes a day 4 times a week, or 17 minutes a day 6 times a week.

Level 3: Walk 30 minutes a day 4 times a week, or 20 minutes a day 6 times a week.

Level 4: Walk 35 minutes a day 4 times a week, or 23 minutes a day 6 times a week.

Level 5: Walk 40 minutes a day 4 times a week, or 26 minutes a day 6 times a week.

Level 6: Walk 45 minutes a day 4 times a week, or 30 minutes a day 6 times a week.

For those people who find that as they walk their heart rate is below their target zone.

TABLE 3. STARTER PROGRAM B

Level 1: Walk 10 minutes a day 3 to 4 times a week.
Level 2: Walk 12 minutes a day 3 to 4 times a week.
Level 3: Walk 14 minutes a day 3 to 4 times a week.
Level 4: Walk 16 minutes a day 3 to 4 times a week.
Level 5: Walk 18 minutes a day 3 to 4 times a week.
Level 6: Walk 20 minutes a day 3 to 4 times a week.

This program is for those people who find that as they walk their heart rate is in their target zone.

If you find this program (Program A) too difficult, walk 10 or five minutes or even less. Once you are able to walk 20 minutes a day four days a week, or 15

minutes a day six times a week, you have reached
Level 1. Stay at this level for at least one week. Then
go to Level 2 and stay there for at least a week, and so
on through the program. So always listen to your
body. You may feel more comfortable spending two
weeks at each level, or maybe a week at one level and
two weeks at another. Whatever works best for you is
fine as long as you spend at least a week at each level.

If you find that you reach your target heart rate
range even when you walk at a fairly slow pace, you
should use Program B (Table 3). If the 10 minutes a
day three or four times a week seems too difficult (if
you are out of breath, etc.), walk only five minutes a
day or less. Some emphysema patients walk only one
minute at the start. You must be the judge.

Some people may think the Starter Program is too
basic, not hard enough. We don't agree. Most people
"attack" a fitness program, and after a few weeks, they
quit. Remember, your primary purpose should be to
get motivated to exercise on a regular basis and keep
at it. Anybody can start an exercise program, but not
everyone can stay at it. So follow these directions and
stay with one of the Starter Programs. Do not jump
ahead.

Don't worry about the speed of your walks. Just
walk for time. As you walk, you may want to take your
pulse. If it's below your target heart rate range, that's
all right for the Starter Program. If it exceeds your
target heart rate range, slow down. And don't worry
about the number of miles you cover. Most people will
cover a mile in 20 minutes; some will be slower, and
some faster. Mileage is not important.

Making Progress

Once you complete the Starter Program, you are ready
for bigger and better things. Now it's time to progress

to the CONSUMER GUIDE ® Walking Program. The Walking Programs are described in Tables 4 and 5.

TABLE 4. WALKING PROGRAM A

If you find your walking puts your heart rate in target heart rate range, then follow this program.

Levels 1-6: See Starter Program B.
Level 7: Walk 22 minutes 3 to 4 times a week.
Level 8: Walk 24 minutes 3 to 4 times a week.
Level 9: Walk 26 minutes 3 to 4 times a week.
Level 10: Walk 28 minutes 3 to 4 times a week.
Level 11: Walk 30 minutes 3 to 4 times a week.
Level 12: Walk 33 minutes 3 to 4 times a week.
Level 13: Walk 36 minutes 3 to 4 times a week.
Level 14: Walk 39 minutes 3 to 4 times a week.
Level 15: Walk 42 minutes 3 to 4 times a week.
Level 16: Walk 45 minutes 3 to 4 times a week.
Level 17: Walk 48 minutes 3 to 4 times a week.
Level 18: Walk 51 minutes 3 to 4 times a week.
Level 19: Walk 54 minutes 3 to 4 times a week.
Level 20: Walk 57 minutes 3 to 4 times a week.
Level 21: Walk 60 minutes 3 to 4 times a week.

Note: The levels that are illustrated on both Programs A and B are guidelines. If at any time the exercise seems excessive or your body is rebelling, cut back. The charts are guidelines at best.

Spend a minimum of one week at each level.

TABLE 5. WALKING PROGRAM B

If your heart rate is below the target heart rate range as you walk, use this chart.

Levels 1-6: See Starter Program A.
Level 7: Walk 50 minutes 4 times a week, or 33 minutes 6 times a week.
Level 8: Walk 55 minutes 4 times a week, or 36 minutes 6 times a week.
Level 9: Walk 60 minutes 4 times a week, or 40 minutes 6 times a week.

Level 10: Walk 65 minutes 4 times a week, or 43 minutes 6 times a week.

Level 11: Walk 70 minutes 4 times a week, or 47 minutes 6 times a week.

Level 12: Walk 75 minutes 4 times a week, or 50 minutes 6 times a week.

Level 13: Walk 80 minutes 4 times a week, or 53 minutes 6 times a week.

Level 14: Walk 85 minutes 4 times a week, or 57 minutes 6 times a week.

Level 15: Walk 90 minutes 4 times a week, or 60 minutes 6 times a week.

Level 16: Walk 95 minutes 4 times a week, or 63 minutes 6 times a week.

Level 17: Walk 100 minutes 4 times a week, or 67 minutes 6 times a week.

Level 18: Walk 105 minutes 4 times a week, or 70 minutes 6 times a week.

Level 19: Walk 110 minutes 4 times a week, or 73 minutes 6 times a week.

Level 20: Walk 115 minutes 4 times a week, or 77 minutes 6 times a week.

Level 21: Walk 120 minutes 4 times a week, or 80 minutes 6 times a week.

Note: Some people find that two hours of walking is a little too much. So we advocate going 80 minutes 6 times a week. Also our experience with walkers shows that when you are not walking at target heart rate levels, 4 times a week or more—not 3—seems to be the best number of days to exercise.

Spend a minimum of one week at each level.

How far you go up on the charts depends on your fitness goals. If you want to improve your physical fitness levels, then you should progress up to Levels 7 to 11, three times a week. If you're interested in weight control and percentage of body fat, your minimum is Level 11, four times a week. If you are interested in reducing cholesterol and triglycerides, then your minimum is Levels 11 through 16, four times a week. If you're interested in possibly experiencing the walker's feeling of euphoria, try Levels 16 to 21.

Walking will allow your heart rate to get up to your target heart rate range. Of course, as you improve, you must walk faster to keep it at that level. Most of you can't shuffle along and expect to reach 70 to 85 percent of your maximum heart rate. You'll have to walk at a good clip. If that is uncomfortable, use Program B. Here you walk longer at a lower pulse rate. This is especially beneficial to the person who is just beginning to exercise after a long layoff.

The following is a good rule of thumb. If you are unable to work at your target level, double the number of minutes you walk. For example, if you want to do 30 minutes of target heart rate exercise and find that you can't get your heart rate up that high, go to 60 minutes or more. It's a fair compromise. And that's exactly what the two walking programs are. They have been adjusted so that you can walk at a level suitable for you. Just remember: listen to your body.

How long and how often you walk depends upon your fitness objectives.

If you're interested in improving your fitness level, you should walk at 70 to 85 percent of your maximum heart rate for at least 20 minutes (15 minutes in a pinch) three times a week. As you start to improve, you may want to work up to about 30 minutes.

If you want to lose weight and fat, walk at 70 to 85 percent of your maximum heart rate for 30 minutes or longer at least four times a week.

If you want to reduce coronary heart disease risk factors like cholesterols and triglycerides (increase the number of high-density lipoproteins), walk at 70 to 85 percent of your maximum heart rate for 30 to 45 minutes or more, four or more times a week.

To help yourself mentally reduce depression and anxiety, work at 70 to 85 percent of your maximum for 45 minutes to an hour, three or more times a week.

To reduce blood pressure, the answer is not quite clear. But the best advice seems to be: Don't worry so much about target heart rates unless you can exercise at that level comfortably. Exercise slowly for at least 30 minutes, five or more times a week.

When to Walk and What to Wear

Listen to your biological clock. Don't try to force yourself into a mold. It won't work. Be specific. Know yourself. If you're an owl, exercise in the evening. If you're a lark, do it in the morning. If the afternoon is your time of day, do it then. Whatever time is appropriate, make sure to give yourself a time commitment. You must be willing to set aside a certain period of time each day or every other day. At first a little experimenting may be necessary to find out what works best for you.

But whatever you do, don't worry about taking the time. You're doing something positive for your body, and it will make you feel better—more productive and more alive. All you are taking is about 4 percent of your day.

The most important equipment you will own when walking are your shoes. You can cover just as much territory in old cut-off shorts and a T-shirt as you can in an expensive designer's outfit. But a good pair of shoes spells the difference between pain and comfort—success and failure.

Your feet take a lot of punishment when you walk and protecting them helps you avoid injuries. When they first begin, walkers think any old shoe will do. They are convinced the expensive running shoes are overrated. This is not so. If you follow this advice, you'll walk without pain. Good shoes are essential. (Of course, there are exceptions. The mountain people of the Andes have gnarled feet that are exceptionally wide. Their feet have so many blood vessels that they are almost immune to the cold. They can walk barefoot on the snow! They can walk for long periods of time across rocky crevices, extremely hard trails, and knife-sharp rocks. But most of us have tender feet.)

Walkers tend to have the same kind of foot problems that runners have. When they use tennis or basketball shoes, they're headed for trouble. Once a person starts to go beyond a half hour of walking daily, he needs a shoe that gives good support. Some people encounter problems at lower levels. So if you're serious about fitness and are going to walk, get a good pair of running shoes. You might ask: Why running shoes for walking? The answer is simple. Running shoes provide the support, protection, comfort, and cushioning that your feet will need for walking on all kinds of surfaces. And you do need support for all the walking you'll be doing. Each mile you walk, your foot hits the ground about 400 times. In a four-mile walk, that's about 1,600 times. If you weigh 200 pounds, each foot receives a total impact of 320,000 pounds—or 160 tons. That's a lot of pounding on your feet, legs, and hips. You'll need support for your feet. You're going to need shoes which will cost you between $20 and somewhat more than $40.

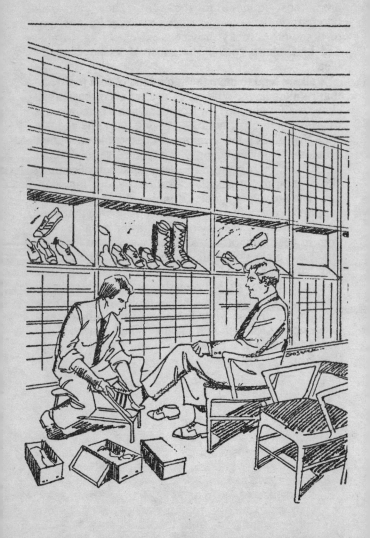

RATING THE SHOES

GENERALLY, SHOES FOR RUNNERS ARE BEST. HERE'S HOW TO SELECT A PAIR.

Your feet will probably be two of the first parts of your body to feel the ill effects of poor walking technique because of their proximity to the ground.

Think about the shoes you're wearing now, or the ones you'll put on tomorrow. Unless they're brand-new, you probably don't notice how they feel on your feet, since they don't pinch or rub you the wrong way. But do you think you could walk a couple of miles in them without suffering? If you've ever had to walk long distances without advance warning (your car broke down on a lonely stretch of road, or you mistakenly got out of the cab at the wrong airline terminal), you know how painful it can be to walk in shoes that do not fit exactly right.

In this chapter we discuss five types of shoes: the conventional "fashion" shoe like the ones you probably wear to work; the shoe with the "negative-heel" design; hiking boots; some new shoes designed especially for people who walk a great deal; and running shoes. We believe running shoes are best for use by persons following a specific walking program.

Those of you who decide to walk to and from work as part of your walking program may not want to wear running shoes and carry your work shoes as you walk. You might try to walk in your work shoes. Is this all right?

To answer that question, we talked with Dr. Harry Hlavac, podiatrist and author of *The Foot Book*. His premise is simple: "If you are walking comfortably in your shoes—no matter what the style—and not experiencing any blisters, irritation, pain, or fatigue, stay with that shoe. There is no reason to change." In other words, leave well enough alone. If you experience pain, fatigue, irritation, blisters, or calluses, you must look elsewhere. You must use great care in selecting a shoe. Dr. Lloyd Nesbitt, Executive Secretary for the Canadian Podiatric Sports Medicine Academy in Toronto, summarized shoe selection this way:

> The shoes you select are to have cushioning such as crepe soles. The cushioned sole lessens the shock that's transmitted up the legs when walking on concrete. Make sure there is ample room in the toe box so that your toes can wiggle a bit. Your foot shouldn't slide from side to side, but there should be room so there is no tightness on the edge of the foot. Narrow, pointed fashion toes are out. The back side of the heels—the heel counters—are to offer good support to the heel. These counters are to be fairly firm. The sole is to flex at the ball of the foot. If it does not flex here you're going to get pains in your Achilles tendon. On the other hand, the sole should not flex in the mid part. There is to be some good support along the sides of the shoes. But the main thing is a cushioned sole. That makes the difference when you're walking long distances.

Concerning the heels, Hlavac says, "The heel elevation should be one-half to three-quarter inch above the sole. Going over two inches in heel height can cause the tendons around the lower legs and feet to overwork."

Hlavac offers some more advice. "Look for a real leather shoe rather than any kind of patent leather or synthetics," he says. "They don't breathe the same way. When you're fitted for shoes be fitted standing as well as sitting. And if one foot is larger than the other, fit the larger foot and use some type of filler for the smaller foot."

Neither doctor would recommend a particular brand of shoe, since many companies are now coming out with good shoes that meet these requirements. It's difficult to recommend one over all the rest, but Hlavac and Nesbitt say that an oxford-type shoe that gives you support around the instep and allows freedom in the toes is better than a slip-on.

The doctors make one more important point. Many people, they say, feel that shoes cause the problem, and if they wear the right shoe everything will be fine. But the problem is poor foot structure. This means problems can occur regardless of the shoe. You have to control the way your foot functions in the shoe. A lot of people have bone calluses in certain areas. Calluses indicate an imbalance. So if you're getting calluses or your feet and your lower legs are hurting, you should see a podiatrist who may recommend an orthotic. Shoes don't cause bunions; you get them because your foot functions incorrectly.

Nesbitt says it is easy to tell whether your shoe is living up to expectations. "Continual pain or aching in the morning when you get up or pain in the lower legs, knees, heels, or arches after walking or standing a long period of time are the main warning signs. So are calluses. One more thing: if your toes are curled, these are indications that something's wrong."

In summary, if you don't have any problems with your feet, don't worry. But if you start to experience calluses, pain, fatigue, and a whole host of other foot and leg problems, go over these recommendations: the heels of your shoes are to be one-half to three-quarter inch high; a crepe sole is best, but if it isn't crepe, then some similar type of cushioning sole is satisfactory; the shoes should be stiff in the shank and flexible at the ball of the foot; toe room must be adequate, and the heel counter must be firm; the preferred fabric for the shoe is real leather; the shoes must be known to fit properly before you buy them; see a doctor or podiatrist if you're still having problems, since an orthotic may be necessary.

Shoes with negative heels are either good or bad for you, depending on which authority you ask. Negative-heel shoes are a very peculiar style of footwear, easily distinguishable by a thick contoured sole that gently slopes downward from the toe to a lowered heel.

Some podiatrists believe the heavy construction and lack of flexibility of negative-heel shoes restrict the motion of the foot. Others warn that the rigid contours of the arch make the shoe uncomfortable for persons with very flat feet or extremely high arches. And still other authorities argue that the negative heel throws the entire body off balance. Exponents of the negative-heel shoe claim the lower heel tends to improve posture. They say slipping the weight back onto the heel causes the wearer to stand more erect.

Nesbitt doesn't recommend this type of shoe. He did a study on these shoes and found that they take some pressure off the ball of the foot. So if you have calluses on your feet, the negative-heel shoe may be helpful. But for people who are used to wearing shoes with high heels, trouble may lie ahead. Achilles tendons can become contracted and shortened as a result of the wearing of high-heeled boots or shoes. A switch to negative-heel shoes can cause a bit of pain. To add to the problem, Nesbitt says, "it's not normal for you to have a great deal of pressure on your heel. For a lot of people, like diabetics, it could be somewhat dangerous. To add to the problem, going up hills causes even more stress."

Hlavac, however, has other ideas. He supports the negative-heel concept and finds that these shoes are desirable for many people.

Any shoes—particularly negative-heel shoes—require

some breaking in. That means two to four weeks of adjustment, a gradual increase in wearing time: one hour the first day, and one hour added every one to three days. During this period, you may have heel pain and mild stiffness or cramps in the calves. Don't be discouraged this early in the game. But if you still feel the sensation after one month's time, take the hint. The negative-heel shoe may not be for you.

So far we've discussed only the shoes that would be used by persons who walk in urban or suburban areas. But what about those of you who may wish to do your walking in the bush? Hiking boots are a necessity. Some people have walked to the tops of mountains in running shoes, but we can't recommend that. If you plan to do any strenuous hiking, you should choose boots, and choose them carefully.

Although all hiking boots tend to look pretty much alike, they can vary significantly. Pay attention to the total weight of the boot. For the average male, boots should weigh about four to five pounds; for the average female, about a half pound less. If the boots are too light, your feet may get banged up. If your boots are too heavy, your legs will suffer from lifting unnecessary extra pounds hour after hour. Generally, if you're going to walk on the road, through the bush, and up mountains, the most versatile model will be what is called a medium-weight hiking (or trail) boot. It may also be called a lightweight climbing boot. (Be wary of "climbing boots": they may not be suitable for prolonged walking.)

Boots should have a hard toe, a rubber-lug sole, padding around the instep and ankle, and uppers that reach at least two inches above your ankle. The upper should be made of good leather. The fewer the seams in the uppers, the more rugged the boot.

Find a store with a salesperson you feel you can trust. Ask a few questions. If you seem to be getting reasonable answers, you can proceed.

Once you've selected your boots, you'll have to

spend some time breaking them in. Wear them around the house and on short walks prior to wearing them for any extended period of time. One week is not enough. It will take you a good month or more to break them in properly. The length of time is contingent upon how much you walk.

Running Shoes: Best for Walking

Despite the name, running shoes are our recommendation for walkers. Although you may talk to serious runners who'll tell you that you don't have to worry about the quality of your shoes unless you intend to log many miles of walking or running each week, we don't agree. If you want to progress smoothly and without pain, invest in a good pair of running shoes. Cheap shoes may save you money, but high-quality shoes will save your feet.

Finding the right shoe can be a bit complicated. There are so many brands on the market that it's difficult to choose. Personal preference plays a big role. What works for one person may not work for another. It comes down to this: if the shoe you have works for you, stay with it. When problems occur, look for common-sense solutions.

The following are CONSUMER GUIDE®'s suggestions of factors to consider when shopping for running-walking shoes. We believe you ought to familiarize yourself with these factors and how they can affect your walking comfort.

Fit. You, not the experts, will be wearing the shoes. So no matter how marvelous the design, if it isn't right for you, it's a waste of money. Your feet, like your fingerprints, are individual. You should make your selection with that in mind.

Begin by drawing an outline of your feet. Place each foot on a piece of paper and draw around it. (The lead of the pencil should follow the curvature of your instep.) Since one foot may be larger than the other, it's a good idea to trace both. When you go to the store, compare the bottom of each shoe to your tracing. How closely do the shoes conform to your feet? Are they wide enough across the ball and the toe? Are they long enough?

When trying on shoes, wear the socks that you will use when walking. If you plan to wear two pairs of socks, as many walkers do, wear both.

Check the toe area with special care. When you walk, your foot will slide forward inside the shoe. Allow about half an inch between your toe and the front of the shoe. Too snug a fit can cause undue pressure, blisters, black toes, and corns. Be sure that your toes have enough room to spread out a little bit. Cramped toes can cause problems.

Lacing. Currently there are three lacing patterns used in shoes. The most common is the U-throat or U-box, which is a full lacing pattern down to the toes in the shape of a U, much like the lacing pattern found on most dress shoes. The vamp, or bulcher, pattern runs across the instep area of the foot and does not go all the way down to the toes. Recently, some shoe manufacturers have emphasized the speed-lacing arrangement. Here the laces pass through plastic or metal rings so the lace does not snag on the material on the shoe's upper when they are being tied. Many U-box or bulcher patterns incorporate speed lacing.

Support. Because your foot hits the ground so many times during the course of a walk, good support is a must. Most shoes designed for walking or running offer some measure of support, but they may not be sufficient for you. If the arch support in an otherwise excellent shoe seems inadequate, you can add foam rubber supports yourself. These inserts are readily available. Good built-in support is preferable, however.

Weight. Ordinary running shoes vary considerably (up to 25 percent) in weight. Weight can be a factor if you plan to run, but it isn't an important consideration for walking.

Flexibility. This is one of the more important factors in judging a shoe. Many injuries are caused by shoes that are too stiff. Unless the sole bends easily, your feet will suffer. Bend the shoe back and forth to test pliability. The foresole must flex. If the sole at the ball of the foot is too stiff, then the Achilles tendon will be overstressed. The stress occurs because the leg works hard to bend the sole at the ball of the foot. If you weigh 200 pounds or more, you'll want more cushioning than sole flexibility. A shoe should not be flexible at the midsole or under the arch. If it is, the bottom of the foot will suffer from lack of support, and plantar fasciitis (a strain or partial rupture of the ligament that runs from the ball to the heel of the foot) will result.

Sole. All soles are made of rubber. They vary greatly in design. The sole must provide protection and cushioning while remaining flexible—no easy thing to accomplish. Most manufacturers solve the problem by providing double soles: a tough outer layer to resist impact; and one or more softer layers inside to cushion the feet and absorb shocks. This combination is definitely better than either hard or soft soles alone.

There also are distinctive tread designs. The trend today is toward the "waffle" tread, which is a series of raised grippers designed to provide greater traction. A number of patterns including square, round, star-shaped, and triangular grippers are offered by different companies. Because the shock of impact is born by the grippers rather than by the whole foot, the waffle tread probably provides more cushioning than a flat tread. But pending further evidence, we believe that tread design is largely a matter of personal preference.

Heel. A moderately elevated heel is best. The shoe should place the heel of the foot higher than the front of the foot. Measure the forefoot thickness at the ball of the foot, and measure the shoe's heel height at the point of maximum thickness of the sole, where it meets the heel of the foot. *Runner's World* magazine says, "A shoe that has a forefoot sole thickness of 14mm should have roughly 26–29mm thickness in the heel area, or 12–16mm more in the heel than in the forefoot."

The shoe should hold the heel of the foot snugly without discomfort. Make sure that the top of the heel hits the back of your foot at a comfortable level. If it is too low, there will not be enough support; if it is extremely high, you may develop blisters or Achilles tendon problems. Compare the depth of the running shoe's heel with that of your regular shoes. The heel counter, the piece on the back of the shoe that supports the heel and Achilles tendon, should be firm and comfortable. The counter should be firm, and the heel tabs should be of adequate height to help stabilize the heel during contact with the ground. It should not be so high as to become a source of chafing itself. The heel width is measured at the widest point from one side of the ankle pad to the other.

Toe box. The toe box design is extremely important. When you're walking downhill, your feet are forced forward in the shoes, so there should be at least a half inch of space between the tip of the longest toe and the inside surface of the front of the shoe. Most importantly, the toe box should be high enough to allow the toes to move freely. If the toe box is too low, the tops of the shoes will rub the tops of the toes and cause black toenails, blisters, and other toe problems. The toe box height should be about 1.2 inches. The toe box height is usually measured about one inch back from the inside top of the shoe.

Uppers. The uppers are the part of the shoe that gives it its distinctive appearance. Resist the temptation to judge a shoe by its color or sportiness. Function is more important. The upper must be firm enough to stabilize the foot and soft enough on the inside so that it doesn't irritate the foot. Avoid shoes with thick seams that may chafe.

Uppers are made of nylon, leather, or combinations of materials. Usually, nylon uppers are best because they are light, permit good air circulation, and are easy to clean. Leather is preferable if you plan to walk a lot in inclement weather.

If you can afford it, buy two pairs of shoes. You might prefer to have one pair for ordinary walking and one pair for bad-weather walking. The extra pair is really a luxury rather than a necessity, however.

It is important to purchase new shoes before the old ones are completely worn out. Wear the new ones on shorter walks to break them in. By the time your old ones are ready to be discarded, the new ones will be comfortable.

COPING WITH PAIN

A FEW ACHES AND PAINS ARE OK—JUST LISTEN TO YOUR BODY.

We've said repeatedly that a well-designed walking program should enable you to enjoy all the benefits of the "training effect" without pain. However, no matter how carefully you follow the CONSUMER GUIDE® Walking Program, you probably will experience a few little aches and pains—simply because you'll be asking your body to do things that it might not have done for years.

We have included this chapter on coping with pain because we don't want a few minor physical discomforts to discourage you from walking. Here we'll explain the types of pain you may encounter and tell you how to alleviate them. As you continue to walk, you will undoubtedly gather your own little private collection of twinges and throbs—"body noises" that will be completely new to you. You are the best judge of what they mean, so pay attention to them. Most of the time your pain will be caused by improper walking technique, poor walking surfaces or shoes, and too much walking too soon.

Often the solution is so simple that you miss it. For example, several members of a walking class complained of continual pain in their left knees. Nothing seemed to help—shoes, physicians, taping. Some of the people had been walking on a banked track; others

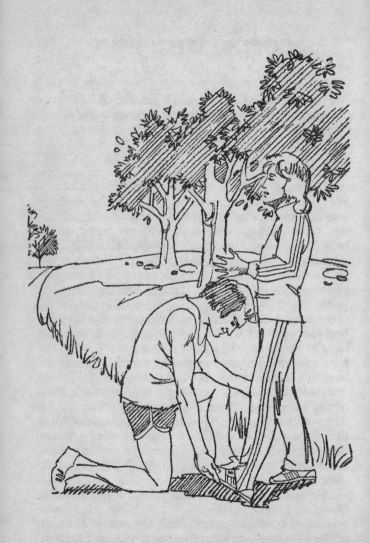

on the banked edge of the road. Suddenly, their instructor asked them to change directions frequently. That way the same leg would not always be on the down side of the bank. It worked like magic. Their pain disappeared almost immediately. The slant of the road and the bank of the track had gradually created an imbalance in their walking style and a strain on their left knees. It isn't always this simple, but this case shows how many times the solution can be found by a little self-analysis and imagination. Everyone will go through pain, more or less. That's one reason why you'll want to ask other walkers what they have experienced. Most of the solutions are just plain common sense.

The ironic thing about walking is that those organs we mainly want to exercise, the heart and lungs, are not the chief source of most of our pain. Instead it's our feet, ankles, legs, and other bones and muscles, which have to work so hard to exercise the heart and lungs, that cause the troubles.

If you want to minimize the amount of pain, you should do three things: (1) take good care of your feet; (2) strengthen the muscles, ligaments, tendons, and joints of the feet, legs, and abdomen; and (3) develop flexibility in the body's muscular system.

Conditioning of your muscles, ligaments, joints, and tendons is a process that will take place naturally and automatically as you walk. But you can help it along by supplementing your walking with calisthenics or other exercises that will develop strength and flexibility. These calisthenics do not benefit the heart and lungs, but they help the body gain more from aerobic exercise. If your muscles and joints are conditioned to work under great stress with a minimum of pain, you are ahead of the game. If not, exercise will give you the conditioning you need.

If you set up a regular exercise program for yourself to parallel your walking program, be sure it is broad and thorough enough to condition all parts of your body. The legs, ankles, and feet are more directly involved in walking than anything else. But you don't want to shortchange the upper part of your body. Refer to our chapter on additional exercises for more information.

From the Ground Up

The following is a summary of the types of aches and pains walkers sometimes feel. We'll begin at the bottom, discussing minor ailments of the feet, then move on up until we reach the chest, where pains can be especially troubling.

The toes. Most pain felt in the toes results from poorly fitted walking shoes. When you try on a new pair of walking shoes, be sure they fit well in the toe. Shoe widths are measured across the widest part of the foot sole, and sometimes tend to taper too drastically in the toe area. Other brands may be too wide there for your particular foot. Make sure the fit is right for you. The size of a walking shoe doesn't really tell you whether it will fit your foot. The shape of your foot finally determines the shoe you should choose for maximum comfort. Select a design that matches your foot as closely as possible. (See our chapter on shoe ratings for some helpful suggestions.)

Few things are more aggravating to a walker than toenails that cut into the flesh of the toes every time the foot comes down against the ground. The solution is simple: keep your toenails trimmed, especially at the corners.

In the foot's longest bones, the metatarsals, the stress of walking can produce fractures so small they may not be visible on an x-ray. Normally they will not have to be splinted or put into a cast. They simply heal by themselves. But it takes time, maybe a month or two, even if you do not subject them to severe strain. This doesn't mean you have to interrupt your walking program while they heal. But during this time it would be wise to walk on very soft surfaces at a reduced pace and for shorter distances.

Morton's Foot. This is not a disease, but a matter of bone structure. Normally the big toe is the longest. People who have Morton's Foot, however, have big toes that are unusually short, and the second toe is longer than the first. This condition upsets normal balance, and the weight stress falls toward the inside arch. Although many people who have Morton's Foot do not experience specific problems, others develop calluses and strains on the foot and leg.

Usually this can be corrected by wearing a special shoe insert called an orthodic, and shoes with roomy toe areas that permit the foot to slide forward without putting pressure on the ends of the toes. If you have foot pain and Morton's Foot, see a podiatrist.

Blisters. These are common ailments. Regardless of the type of shoe worn and the protective measures taken, foot blisters continue to be a problem for many people. They become a major problem only when they are severe enough to affect the quantity and quality of walking. Problems also occur when infection develops.

Foot blisters are caused by heat. They are really burns produced by friction. The best way to prevent blisters is to prevent the friction that causes them. Here are some recommendations.

1. Buy high-quality shoes and make sure they fit properly.
2. Take good care of your shoes. Don't allow them to get brittle so that "hot spots" develop.
3. Break in new shoes before walking very far. A good idea is to first wear the shoes around the house for a few minutes each day. As they begin to soften, wear them for walking short dis-

tances (10 to 20 minutes). As they start to break in, you can wear them for longer distances.

4. Wear socks to help prevent blisters. The socks should be clean and fit snugly.

When a blister does develop, prevent infection by keeping the area clean. Do not puncture small blisters immediately. If you do puncture a blister once it has grown larger, puncture it with a sterile needle to release the fluid, squeezing gently with sterile gauze. Do not remove the skin. Place a pad of gauze and, possibly, foam rubber over the open blister. Continue to walk if you can do so without significant pain. Consult your physician or podiatrist at the first sign of infection or complications.

Walker's heel. This is a term some people use to describe a group of heel problems that include bone bruises and heel spurs (painful bony growths on the heel bone itself). These ailments are normally caused by walking on a hard surface, stepping on sharp objects with force enough to cause a bruise, or wearing poorly designed walking shoes. These complaints don't lend themselves to a quick cure. Rest is good for them, but not always desirable for the person who wants to maintain his or her conditioning.

As far as treatment is concerned, the best thing is a heel "donut." This is nothing more than a foam pad with a hole cut in it. You can place the foam pad over the bone spur with the sensitive spot protruding through the hole. Then tape the donut to your foot. Many people have had excellent success with this. One gentleman, 72 years of age, complained of a heel bruise. Three doctors recommended surgery, but Charles T. Kuntzleman suggested that he try the donut before making a final decision on surgery. In a matter of weeks, he was pain-free. Today, six years later, he is still walking and no longer has a walker's heel. Anytime he feels a sensitivity in his heel, he wears a donut for a few days and it disappears.

This even works for nonwalkers. George is a truck driver. He had to get in and out of his truck 20 to 50 times a day. Over the years he developed a severe spur on the top of his foot. He had surgery twice, and each time the spur came back. When it started to appear the third time, his wife, Kuntzleman's secretary, asked what George could do. Kuntzleman again suggested a donut. To George's surprise, the bone spur disappeared, and surgery was not necessary. That was five years ago, and the spur hasn't reappeared.

If this doesn't work for you, see a podiatrist.

Achilles tendon injuries. The Achilles tendon is the thick tendon at the back of the leg that connects the heel and foot to the back of the calf muscles. It controls the hinge-like action of the ankle with every walking step and therefore does a lot of work during a walk. Achilles tendon injuries are extremely debilitating. Some people have said, in fact, that once you have an Achilles problem, you will always have a problem.

Sports medicine experts have identified three types of problems with the Achilles tendon. The first is tendinitis, which is an inflammation of the tendon. The second is a partial rupture, which is a tearing of the tendon fibers. The third is a complete rupture, or a complete break, of the tendon itself. The last two are not common to most walkers.

Tendinitis is usually caused by a sudden change in routine, such as different types of shoes, or walking on grass and then switching to cinders, or going from one type of training to another. Symptoms of tendinitis are pain and stiffness an hour or so following activity, slight swelling, pain on contraction and stretching of the calf muscles, and tenderness when squeezing pressure is applied at the tendon's narrowest point. Walking becomes very difficult and painful.

Tendons also become inflamed and swollen when

they are constricted by equipment. If you feel pain in your Achilles tendon, your walking shoes could be the culprit. The heels may be too low or too hard, or the backs may be too tight, straining or crowding the tendon. Perhaps the arch support in the shoes is not adequate. Tendinitis can also be caused by years of wearing heeled shoes. The heels favored by Americans shorten the Achilles tendons and make them less flexible. The very act of walking often tightens these tendons even more, just as it develops the muscles of the legs. This is one reason why stretching exercises are important to the walker. They limber up the tendons and counteract the effects of walking and the wearing of heels.

Self-treatment of tendinitis can be summarized in a few sentences. If it hurts you, put cold water or ice on the injured area. Reduce your activity until what pain there is isn't intolerable. Slow down or stop if pain gets worse while exercising. In simple terms, if you're not hurting, you probably aren't hurting yourself.

When you first injure your Achilles tendon, stretching should be avoided at all costs. Over-stretching led to the problem in the first place. Walk on flat, smooth, straight surfaces. Do not do any fast walking. As long as there is tendon inflammation and pain, ice or cold water after each walking session may be helpful. But this will not really cure the injury—it simply helps you endure the pain.

To prevent Achilles tendinitis from developing, make sure that you do plenty of stretching in your warm-ups. Suggested stretching exercises include standing on the heels of the feet, drawing the toes up as far as possible, or putting your toes on a two-inch board and stretching the heel downward. Another good idea is to walk barefooted whenever possible.

Also avoid sudden and violent changes in routine: for example, walking on a level surface and then suddenly changing to walking on hills; walking on a track and then suddenly switching to a road; or walking short distances and then suddenly walking long distances.

Be careful about your shoes. For years Charles T. Kuntzleman believed that sore calves were a part of running. Then one day he was told that a higher heel would help. He tried it and liked it. Kuntzleman now has no more calf pain. The same applies to walkers.

Shin splints. Shin splints are a pain on the front of the shin. If you have a shin splint you will feel pain in the lower leg when you put weight on your foot. You'll probably also find that your shin is tender to the touch. When you run your fingers along the shin, you may feel a roughened area along the bone.

Although the name implies a splintering or damage to the shin bone, it may be any of several conditions. Here are a few possibilities: (1) You may have a muscle imbalance caused by a "toeing out" of the feet or other improper body mechanics; (2) there may be a hairline fracture of one of the bones in the lower leg; (3) a muscle spasm may occur because of the swelling of the muscle in the front of the leg; (4) the tendon that is attached to the bone of the lower leg may be inflamed; (5) the same tendon or the muscle may be torn from the bone; (6) the membrane between the two bones of the lower leg may be irritated; (7) your arch may drop somewhat, thereby irritating one or more of the tendons of the lower leg.

You can prevent shin splints by taking care when choosing your footwear and the surfaces you walk on. A good pair of shoes with a rippled sole and heel is probably best. Shoes with cushioned soles are a must. It's also a good idea to have a shoe with a low heel. If possible, switch from a hard to a soft walking surface. A golf course or a local park offers the walker a chance to work out on grass, which is much softer than pavement or a track. If you walk on a track, vary the direction of your walking. Instead of always going counterclockwise, walk clockwise on alternate days so that you do not always place stress on the inside of the same leg as you go around the turns.

Also try to avoid walking on your toes. This has been cited as one of the causes of shin splints. Put a sponge heel pad in the heel section of your shoe to help absorb some of the stress from walking on harder surfaces. You can also try placing a molded crest under the toes.

To prevent shin splints from occurring, it's also a good idea to condition the muscles in the front of the leg. Walking does a great deal to strengthen the muscles in the back of the leg. And as a result, muscle imbalance occurs. The muscles in the back of the leg become a lot stronger than the ones in the front, and this sets you up for shin splints. To compensate, you'll want to strengthen the muscles in the front. Doing foot flexors with weights or isometric exercises can help. Flex your foot up and down against resistance. If you don't have weights handy to strap on your feet, sit with your legs dangling, feet not touching the floor, and have a friend hold your feet while you try to pull your toes up. Do this for three sets of 10 each day.

The knee. The knee, the largest and most complicated joint of the body, is a true hinge joint. The two main bones of the joint are the thigh and shin bone. All leg muscles and ligaments, which are essential to the efficient movement and support of the joint, are attached to the thigh and shin bones.

Although the knee is the largest joint in the body, it is vulnerable to injuries, largely because of a poor bone arrangement. Its main support of the joint is from tendons and ligaments, and it has very little defense against a blow from the side. Injuries to the knee joint can be disabling. In some instances, they can keep you from participating in athletics, especially contact sports.

But, despite its vulnerability, your knee can stand a remarkable degree of stress and still work well. It is able to survive even a brutal crush by several 250-pound football players hitting it from different angles—strains beyond the imagination of most people.

On your walk through the neighborhood or along the beach, your knees are not completely safe from stress. Usually knee pains are associated with the kneecap—beneath it or along its sides. Sometimes the kneecap does not move smoothly against the lower end of the thighbone as it should, and the knee becomes increasingly irritated and swollen as you walk. If you have this problem, you may have to limit your walking. But first experiment with different walking methods. Many doctors think this problem may be caused or aggravated by the way your foot strikes the ground. If you walk indoors on a banked track in one direction for long distances, say 20 to 25 laps, your knees may be headed for trouble. Even a subtle slope such as that on a banked road or on a beach may also cause problems.

Many walkers and runners develop a painful affliction called runner's knee in which the kneecap moves from side to side with each step. The reason is most often a foot that collapses when walking. When the foot collapses, the lower leg rotates inward and the kneecap moves to the inside. Repeated foot strikes and a poor foot structure will adversely affect the knee. Treatment usually consists of orthodics to control foot function. It's also important that the participant do leg exercises to strengthen and stretch the muscles on the front of the thighs.

Muscle cramps and spasms. When one of your muscles contracts powerfully and painfully, you have a muscle cramp. The contraction may occur at any time—at rest as well as during activity. Cramps usually occur without warning. Occasionally, however, you may be able to feel one building up.

Among the causes of muscle cramps are fatigue; cold; imbalance of salt, potassium, and water levels; a sharp blow; and overstretching of unconditioned muscles. (The cramps that a person gets when stretching in bed are brought on by a combination of fatigue and overstretching of unconditioned muscles.)

You can probably reduce the chances of muscle cramps by maintaining a proper diet, making sure you warm up properly prior to vigorous activity, and stopping activity before you become extremely fatigued. Tapering off is a good idea.

Once a cramp does occur, it can usually be stopped by stretching the muscle affected and firmly kneeding it. Usually, a sense of tightness or dull pain will follow, making it necessary to apply heat and massage to the area to restore circulation. If you're plagued with frequent cramps, drinking adequate fluid and eating foods high in salt and potassium, along with muscle strengthening and stretching exercises, will usually eliminate the problem.

Sprains and strains. Cramps and spasms are essentially painful contractions of muscle tissue. A strain is a stretching or tearing of a muscle or tendon; a sprain is a stretching or tearing of a ligament. Small blood vessels in the area break and pain develops when the surrounding tissue swells up and overstimulates sensitive nerve endings.

Two common problems are ankle strains and sprains. Obviously, you should watch where you're going. This means that even if you are the casual type and not too finicky about walking on a particular kind of surface, you should at least learn how to pick your way among the potholes and skillfully sidestep any beer cans in your path. If you aren't very good at that and manage to sprain or strain your ankle, you'll have to suspend your walking program until it is healed.

Muscle soreness and stiffness. Even people who have been walking for years complain of regular soreness and stiffness. The pain may occur immediately following the activity or after some delay, usually 24 to 48 hours. Often the discomfort lasts for only a few days, although after periods of severe exercise, it may last for a week. The most commonly affected muscles are the calves and front and back muscles of the thigh.

Medical authorities aren't certain what causes soreness and stiffness. The pain during and immediately following exercise is probably due to waste products formed during exercise and left in the fluid that surrounds the cells. When stiffness occurs approximately 24 to 48 hours after exercise, it may be the result of small muscle tears or localized contractions of muscles.

It is practically impossible to completely avoid muscle soreness and stiffness. But you can reduce the intensity of the pain by planning your conditioning program so that you progress gradually, especially during the early stages. That approach will allow the muscles of the body to adapt themselves to the stress placed upon them. If you become sore and stiff from physical activity, doing some additional light exercises or general activity will often provide temporary relief, though the pain usually returns when you stop. Tapering off will also help to avoid such undesirable aftereffects. Massage will, too.

Back pains. Don't fool around when you get back pains, especially if they are in the lower back. The low back pain can signal a slipped spinal disc. Obviously, back problems cannot be diagnosed on the walking path, but if you have a slipped disc, you'll know it—fast.

Some lower back pains result from exercising after years of relative inactivity. You will have to guess at the seriousness of these pains by the way you feel at the time; that is, how intense they are, how much they cripple you, and so on. In any case, go slow. If for any reason you think further exercise might cause any harm, ask your doctor.

There are, of course, several traditional explanations for back pain. You've probably heard them already, but they're worth repeating. Improper sitting posture can lead to low back problems. As in lifting, the back should be kept erect. Sitting slouched in a chair puts unnecessary tension on the back muscles. Furniture that is constructed without regard for body structure can cause strain, fatigue, and muscle pain. Sitting for prolonged periods of time causes shortening of certain postural muscles, particularly the hamstring muscles. If you sit all day at work, you must do stretching exercises regularly to keep hamstring muscles at their proper length.

A bed that is too soft or sags in the middle is the worst enemy of any back. No matter how you lie on this kind of mattress, your muscles are under constant tension all night long. It is no wonder that these muscles, the spinal erectors being the ones most often affected, are sore in the morning. Many medical experts suggest the use of a board under the mattress to alleviate the condition.

But the real problem is poor fitness; specifically, weak abdominals. At the pelvis, the weight of the upper body is transferred to the lower limbs. The pelvis, or pelvic girdle, is balanced on the rounded heads of the thigh bones. To the pelvis are attached numerous muscles which hold it in place. Some of the muscles involved are the abdominals, hamstrings, gluteals, and hip flexors. An imbalance or weakness in those muscles can lead to pelvic misalignment, which usually causes the pelvis to tilt forward or backward.

If the abdominal muscles which are attached to the front of the pelvis and hold it up are weak, the top of the pelvis will drop and tilt forward. The sacrum (just below the spine) also tilts forward, putting increased tension on the sacroiliac joint and the ligaments located on the front of the lumbar vertebrae. Forward tilt of the pelvis leads to lordosis, or sway back. This is when the "slipped disc" injury most often occurs.

In addition to abdominal weakness, a lack of strength in the gluteals and/or hamstrings can also lead to forward pelvic tilt. While the abdominals stabilize the pelvis by pulling upward on the front, the gluteals and hamstrings contribute to stabilizing by pulling down on the rear of the pelvis.

Exercises must be done to strengthen the abdominals and gluteals. Usually the walking does it for the gluteals. But the abdominal muscles must be conditioned in other ways, such as those described in our chapter on additional exercises.

Quite a few walkers have found that their back pain disappeared after this kind of exercise program; that is, walking and abdominal exercises. But this isn't a miracle cure. On the contrary, you must be extremely cautious. If you have back trouble and do not approach walking with common sense and care, you can make the condition worse.

Side stitch. Side stitch has many names. It is called a pain in the side, a stitch in the side, side ache, or just plain stitch. Sometimes it frightens people because it occurs near the chest area. There are as many explanations of the cause of side stitch as there are names to describe it. But there are probably two basic causes.

The first is improper breathing. This causes spasms in the diaphragm. To reduce the problem, "belly breathing" is suggested. That is, when you inhale, the diaphragm should distend, pushing the abdominal wall out. When you exhale, the diaphragm should be pushed in so that the belly is flattened. It's just the reverse of what you normally do.

The second cause is probably the more common. It's a spasm of the ligaments that are connected to the liver, pancreas, stomach, and intestines. These ligaments are put under stress when you walk vigorously. The bouncing action causes these ligaments to stretch, thereby causing pain. Charles T. Kuntzleman says he has been able to end side stitch by simply gripping his side and pushing it in. In severe cases, you can lie on your back and raise your feet in the air or even try standing on your head or hands. (Kuntzleman says one day in New Orleans, he and his wife were walking quite briskly and she developed a stitch. Belly breathing didn't work, nor did pressing her side. So right on St. Charles Street, Kuntzleman flipped his wife upside down and had her stand on her hands for a few seconds. The pain disappeared, and they returned to a normal pace. That may seem absurd, but it worked. The explanation that a side stitch is caused by repetitive bouncing that strains abdominal ligaments is what gave Kuntzleman the idea. The inverted position, he says, relaxed the ligaments and relieved the spasm.)

There are some other things you can try. Don't eat or drink within three hours before walking; during the attack bend forward, inhale deeply, and push the belly out; if the pain is intolerable, lie flat on your back, raise your legs over your head, and support your hips.

Chest Pain: How Serious Is It?

Any pain in the chest, no matter what its cause, can be troubling—especially if you've reached middle age. Such pain often results in unnecessary concern, because it can be caused by factors that are in no way related to the condition of your heart. However, chest pain should never be ignored or allowed to persist.

Here we'll explain the causes of chest pain—everything from heartburn to heart attacks. We hope this will be able to put your mind at ease about some kinds of chest pain, while inducing you to remain extremely cautious about other kinds.

Kuntzleman often tells the story of one man who'd enrolled in a fitness class he supervised. It serves as an example of how some people go overboard with worry about the health of their heart.

Ten years ago in one of my fitness classes I had a participant named Larry. He was one of my first walkers. Larry experienced chest pain when walking. He tried to ignore the pain, but it was there, big as life, in the middle of his chest. Each time he walked, it reappeared to chill his warm sweat and flash images of a heart attack through his brain. He stopped walking for a month, replacing his morning ritual with calisthenics. But the pain returned when he started walking again. In a panic, he made an appointment with his physician. After all, he reasoned, a million Americans die each year from cardiovascular diseases, and it's not uncommon to read or hear about men in their 50s (like himself), or even 40s, dropping dead from a heart attack. Larry never abused or neglected his body, ate the right foods, didn't smoke or drink, and walked faithfully.

After an hour of numerous tests, the doctor pronounced Larry "fit as a fiddle." The exercise electrocardiogram displayed a sound heart, and the accompanying physical exam described glowing health.

"But what about the pain in my chest, doc?" Larry asked. "It's really there."

"Well," the doctor shrugged, "The only explanation I can give is that it's phychosomatic. The cause of your pain originates in your mind."

Larry returned home, convinced that the doctor was right. His heart was sound and his body was fit. Therefore, the chest pain had to be psychosomatic. Larry reviewed every step of the examination and repeated every word that was said in an effort to totally convince himself that all was well. But he was still worried. Finally he decided to prove his doctor right.

At 6:00 the next morning, Larry was out walking, and as if set off by a precision timepiece, the pain began at 6:10. Larry responded by picking up speed and walking faster and faster until he was exhausted.

In less than a week of walking "through the pain," the chest pain stopped. And it never reappeared.

Although Larry's way of handling chest pain may be unique, his immediate conclusion that the pain was caused by a faulty heart is typical. We are warned so much about heart disease that the slightest twinge in the chest area can conjure up frightening visions of permanent disability, or even death, from cardiovascular disturbances. A seizure in the chest can be, and often is, caused by a cardiovascular disease. But far more often it is caused by a simpler and less damaging ailment, such as heartburn or a strained muscle. Or as in Larry's case, it can be psychosomatic.

Psychosomatic chest pain. An estimated "20 million people in the United States are cardiac patients without heart disease," according to Howard R. and Martha E. Lewis in their book, *Psychosomatics*. According to the authors, these people suffer symptoms that are common to heart disease, such as palpitations, shortness of breath, exhaustion, and chest pain; but the symptoms are really only reactions to stress.

Mind and body are so inseparable that every emotional experience we have is also a physical event. By simply thinking about a problem, you can raise your pulse, cause sweating, bring on headaches and any number of other symptoms. In effect, this is self-inflicted stress, and that stress can cause pain.

A combination of natural and emotional stress factors caused Larry to experience pain in his chest. Some doctors call it a "sympathetic" nervous response. He consciously identified the ache with his heart and unconsciously with walking. So each time he walked, he anticipated pain, and the emotional stress of that fear created the pain.

Researchers have recently discovered that certain events, such as a change of job or a visit of a relative can bring on illness—even the common cold. After the events are resolved—the relative returns home, the new job works out well—the ailments clear up. But according to Thomas H. Holmes writing in *Psychology Today* (April 1972), when researchers started to talk to the patients about those events, the symptoms recurred during the conversation. For example, just talking about one patient's relative was sufficient to give him a runny nose. And for Larry, just thinking he had a bad heart was enough to give him pain when he walked.

It is very difficult to distinguish psychosomatic heart pain from an actual pain. Psychosomatic pain usually is vague. The person "feels" like he has a chest pain, but he can't be specific. Usually the tests given by the doctor also reveal no heart damage or disease.

Muscular causes. Larry's original pain may have had a physical cause. It might have been caused by a muscle spasm. A pulled pectoral (chest muscle) or a strained intercostal (side muscle) can cause a great deal of pain. A pulled muscle produces pain which is felt near the surface, and movements such as swinging the arm across the chest can initiate or worsen the pain. Bruised muscles and ligaments may cause pain during deep breathing, and they normally remain sensitive to touch. Pressure during sleep from a hand, mattress button, or even a wrinkled sheet may aggravate bruised muscles. Pain associated with this kind of condition usually only occurs during a certain motion and when pressure is applied to the area. Rest and time are usually the best treatments.

Heartburn. The pain brought on by indigestion, or heartburn, is frequently confused with heart pain. But it has nothing to do with the heart. Acid from the stomach backs up into the esophagal tube, causing contractions of the circular muscle of the esophagus. Milk or plain water may give temporary relief, but a simple diet of less highly seasoned food is the best prevention. Heartburn is often confused with real heart disease. If you can attribute the pain to a specific food, your worries are over. If you can't, see your doctor.

Angina pectoris. Known as the "cardiac pain of effort," angina pectoris usually develops during exercise, when emotion is high, or after a heavy meal. It is the result of a temporary failure of the coronary arteries to supply enough oxygenated blood to the heart muscle. Such a failure is usually caused by obstructions to coronary circulation.

Almost anyone can experience angina: people who have recovered from a heart attack, people who are going to have an attack, and some people who will never have an attack. The problem is that your heart muscle is simply not getting enough blood and oxygen. See your doctor if you suspect its presence. In all probability he will permit you to walk as long as you can walk without pain. Don't push yourself to exhaustion. Your doctor will probably want you to be very specific about where the pain appears when you're walking (if it does) so he can fully understand your condition.

Angina pain is usually not sharp; it usually is heavy, giving the victim the sensation that he or she is being squeezed or crushed in the center of the chest. The discomfort often spreads to the left shoulder, arm, or hand, where it may be felt as numbness. Pains may occur days, weeks, months, even years apart. The best treatment following an attack is to rest and to avoid excitement and fatigue.

The pains associated with coronary heart disease are varied, yet similar to angina. They may be sharp or mild with a feeling of numbness. A good rule to follow regarding chest pain is that if the pain abruptly ends after exertion, see your physician.

If you experience any of these pains, particularly the kind that cause heavy pressure and radiate up the neck or down the arm, see your doctor. A very heavy pressure, as if someone were sitting on top of your chest; an extreme tightness, like a clenched fist inside the center of your chest; a feeling something like indigestion, a stuffiness high in your stomach or low in your throat, may signal a heart attack. Whenever you have a strong symptom that resembles any one of these, stop walking and get to your doctor.

You may have gone through a stress ECG before you started a walking program and passed it with flying colors. If so, your chances of having this experience are relatively small. But don't become cocky. A stress ECG, like most tests doctors perform on you, is not 100 percent reliable.

In the final analysis, your body, not somebody else's electronic equipment, has the last word. Listen to it.

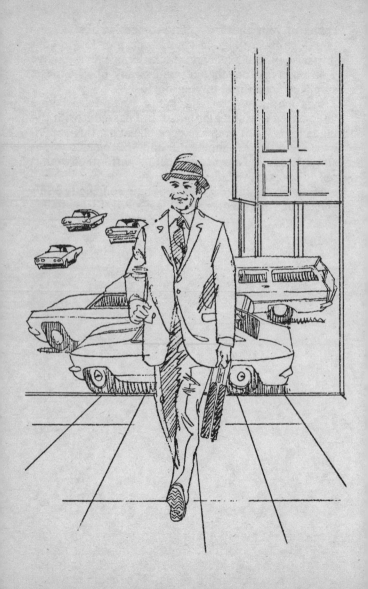

STAYING WITH IT

THERE ARE SOME TRICKS YOU CAN USE TO KEEP YOURSELF INTERESTED.

You're convinced, right? We've succeeded in talking you into beginning a walking program and getting yourself into shape That's great.

However, if you're like many sedentary people who know they ought to be more active, you may already be wondering how long you'll be able to stay with your program of physical conditioning. You may doubt your own stick-to-itiveness. Maybe you're asking yourself: "How long will it be before I lose interest, or develop a blister and give up, or invent any number of other silly excuses for not walking?" Remember Sally?—too hot, too cold, too windy.

Don't let these worries keep you from starting to walk. Begin now, and refer to this chapter whenever you feel a need for another dose of encouragement. We're now going to tell you exactly how to stay with it.

The Proper Attitude

Step One: Set a goal. You're not going to get far without a specific objective. Goals are important in life. They give you something specific to work toward and a way to measure your progress. When you're setting a goal, avoid vague generalizations: "I want to get into shape," or "I want to lose weight." Instead, set precise long-term, intermediate, and short-term goals.

For example, if you want to lose weight, find out what your best weight is and decide how much weight you want to lose in six months or a year. If you want to lose 20 pounds during that period, that is your long-term goal. Your short-term goal might be three pounds by the end of the first month. (Your intermediate goal would be somewhere in between.) Your long-term goal might be 90 minutes of walking a day after 20 weeks. A short-term goal may be 20 minutes of walking a day. An intermediate goal, on the other hand, may be to add one minute of walking a day over the next month.

What kind or how many goals should you set? Take stock of yourself right now. What would you like to do? Whatever it is, write it down now. Even if it seems unrealistic at this time, put it on a sheet of paper or card and save it. These are your long-term goals. Once a week, take out the sheet of paper and look at it. Write down your progress and what seems to be preventing you from achieving everything you want through walking.

Next, you need to plan how you are going to reach those goals. Write it down, and be specific. For example, how many minutes of walking are you going to increase each week to get to your long-term goal? Jot down some motivators you are going to use to help yourself walk.

Finally, make a note of what you'll do today; not tomorrow, but today. Write down how long, at what time, and where you're going to walk. Each morning, as soon as you get up, do the same thing until you reach your long-term goal.

Step Two: Record your progress. For some of us, the thing that makes football, basketball, or ice hockey interesting is the competition. If competition really gets you moving, you can get it from walking. Just use a progress chart. A progress chart lets you compete with yourself. It also tells you and anyone else who looks at it how well you're doing and how close you're getting to your goal. It gives you a feeling of accomplishment.

The chart doesn't have to be complicated. The simplest one is a calendar with the information written in. Many people record their mileage on a map. Your regular walking route may take you around the same section of your neighborhood every day, but you can mark off your distance on a map as though you were walking cross-country. By the end of a year, you may find that you've walked a distance equal to that between San Francisco and San Diego or between New York and Miami. This helps in setting long-term goals, too. For instance, you can promise yourself that you'll walk from Chicago to Dallas this summer.

Step Three: Make a time commitment. Have you ever noticed how easily you slip into routines? Perhaps you always brush your teeth before, not after, you shower in the morning; always put your left, not your right, shoe on first; take the same route to work every day. And have you ever noticed how you tend to feel you've forgotten to do something important if anything should interfere with this strange little ritual? You may find it easy to stay with a walking program if you can allow it to become part of your daily routine— so much a part that you'll feel compelled to walk despite your own excuses for skipping a day. If you can get yourself into the habit of walking at a certain time every day, you'll accept it as part of your regular daily schedule and not just something to do during odd moments.

Whatever you do, don't worry about taking the time. Your co-workers may take a two-hour, three-martini lunch and think nothing of it. And they may cast a scornful eye at you as you go off to take your walk at noon. But you'll be doing something positive for your body, and it will make you feel better, more productive, and more alive.

Step Four: Choose the best time of day. The best time depends on you. Some walkers like to walk early in the morning, some even before daybreak. They seem to like the solitude available at that hour, when the streets are still empty of traffic and people. They can slowly get their minds and bodies going and do a little thinking in the silence. And if they are walking where they can see the horizon, they can savor the exhilarating sight of dawn.

If you do walk before going to work, it is probably a good idea to nibble on something beforehand so your body has the fuel it needs for the walk. There are really no iron-clad rules, but something very light such as a piece of toast and a small glass of orange juice is best.

Some people skip lunch and use the time to walk. It gets them out of the office or house and into a refreshing mid-day break. Other walkers wait until they have left their work, put their jobs behind them, and headed home. A walk at this time provides a nice transition for them, a time to work off some of the day's tensions so that they don't have to carry them into family life.

Late evening seems to appeal to some people as the best time. There is both good news and bad news about walking late in the evening. First, the bad news: when you make walking the last item on your agenda for the day, it often gets treated that way—last. You tend to put other things in place of it. You either forget it, "just don't have the time," or don't have the energy to do it. Now for the good news. When you walk late in the evening, you'll find the walk relaxing. You'll be able to unwind. Some walkers find the late evening walk the best sleeping aid ever invented.

Step Five: Dress the part. If possible, have a special outfit and wear it only for walking. Anything comfortable—an old pair of shorts or jeans and a sweatshirt, for instance—will do. How you look is not the point; it's how you feel. In changing from regular clothes into a "walking outfit," you also psych yourself up for the activity. In effect, you're telling yourself you mean business and really intend to collect your rewards.

Step Six: Think the part. What happens in your head is almost as important as what happens to your body, because if you don't enjoy what you're doing, you'll begin to find reasons for not doing it.

Before you walk, try to get yourself into a positive, active frame of mind. As you walk, be aware of what's happening to your body. Feel your muscles work. Concentrate on the rhythmic flow of your movements. Walking can be a pleasurable sensory experience if you can learn to think of it that way.

Step Seven: Walk with others. If you're married, your spouse has to be on your side. A study conducted at the Heart Disease and Stroke Control Program bears this out. Men in an exercise program did one hour of physical activity three times a week for eight months. If the wife encouraged participation, the individual's attendance was good; if the wife was neutral or had negative feelings about the exercise, attendance was much poorer. The conclusion: the spouse's attitude was critical.

Walking with a friend gives you the advantage of companionship and encouragement. And you will walk more if you have someone to talk to and to keep you company. This is also a good way to assure yourself that you can pass the talk test.

In an investigation conducted at the University of Toronto, scientists reported a greater dropout rate for individual, rather than group, programs: only 47 percent of those on individual programs were still active at 28 weeks, compared with 82 percent of those in the group programs. If you feel your motivation is weak, walk with a partner or with several friends.

Step Eight: Pick a pleasing route. Where you choose to walk is up to you. The range of choices obviously is unlimited—at least as far as space is concerned.

Maybe you're lucky enough to live in a town that

offers not just walking space—every town has that—but different kinds of spaces to make your walks as interesting as possible. You'll soon have your favorite, and you'll probably discover new ones every week. While making discoveries, always consider safety. Traffic must always be taken into account. And some city areas are just not safe enough to walk through at any hour. The best way to protect yourself against these possible dangers is to check over the route you plan to use ahead of time.

When you choose a route, pay close attention to the surface. A lot of walkers say grass is the very best surface for walking. City dwellers can usually find some strip of grass or other unpaved areas to walk on, even if it's only the boulevard along a street. If you can't find a nice, springy green surface to use, pavement is an alternative. One good thing about pavement—you don't have to travel far to find it. But it does have its drawbacks. Most foot and leg problems are either caused or aggravated by walking on hard surfaces like concrete or asphalt. Wearing good, shock-absorbing walking shoes can help avoid this.

If you must use the street instead of the sidewalk, you must be alert for cars. Even if you wear reflective strips on your clothing, you may not be seen by a motorist. Walk as you drive—defensively.

There's another thing you can do to have an enjoyable walk even if you're not surrounded by trees, grass, and fresh country air. Find an old residential area with beautiful homes and meandering streets that can occupy your attention while you walk. Stay away from traffic lights and congested areas where there is a lot of stop-and-go walking. They can cause you to lose momentum and break your stride because you will be concerned about collisions.

Wherever you go, be sure to watch out for dogs. Most walkers have found that the best way to get rid of dogs is to talk sternly to them. Act as if you are their master. Don't show fear. Just speak directly to them, point your finger, and shout.

There are some things to watch out for if you plan to walk in the country. Make sure you're not trespassing. Also, be careful that you don't get carried away by the beauties of nature, the music of the birds, and get lost.

Step Nine: Walk tall. Don't worry about what other people think. As you're walking down Main Street, you may think that everyone is looking at you. So what!—you're doing something good for your body; they're not. You have to learn that some of the stares people are giving you are really nothing more than envy. At least one psychologist has said that the reason he felt people stared at him as he walked was because they wished they had his ambition. People also might be looking at you with admiration.

You may also feel a little embarrassed about walking next to the road. If you do this very often, you'll find that people will ask you questions, such as, "Did your car break down? Can we give you a lift?" You have several alternatives. First, you can tell them, "No thanks, I'm walking." Second, you can tell them, "I only have a few more steps to go." Third, you can pretend you're going shopping. Finally, you can take your dog with you. Everyone knows that a dog needs exercise.

If these don't seem to work, then it may be best to walk where you can't be seen. One couple was so embarrassed about walking outside that they decided to walk in the huge underground parking garage of their apartment complex.

The Walking Commuter

Many walkers we know have managed to work their walking program into their daily commuting. They're proof of what we've been saying throughout this book: walking is the easiest of all exercises to build into your routine.

Bob Rodale, President of Rodale Press, Emmaus, Pennsylvania, lives three miles from his office. In 1968, he started walking to work. It was the only way he could consistently get the exercise he felt he needed. So his program became three miles in the morning and three miles in the evening—in all kinds of weather. Over the years, he has accumulated a wardrobe that makes his walk comfortable: a special rain jacket, walking shoes, knapsack to carry his "homework," and winter garb. He wears a bicyclist's arm lamp so motorists can spot him as he walks home in the evening along a rural road that follows the winding Little Lehigh River. The 45-minute walk in the morning and evening takes a little longer than a car ride, but the rewards, according to Rodale, are well worth it.

Dr. Theodore Klumpp, Chairman of the Board of Winthrop Laboratories, New York City, is a strong advocate of exercise. During his years as a medical student at the Harvard University Fatigue Laboratory, Klumpp saw the benefits of exercise, how it can slow the progress of degenerative diseases, particularly heart disease and diabetes. Convinced that the human body is designed for motion, Klumpp has built walking into his commuting. Each morning he parks his car a little more than a half mile from the Long Island train station and briskly walks the rest of the way. The train stop is a mile from his office, so he walks that distance, too. Then he reverses this pattern in the evening. Klumpp, 75, is also chairman of the board of the Association for Human Development and is associated with many other rehabilitation and human development organizations. He doesn't show any signs of slowing down. The reason, as he puts it, for his good health, vigor and longevity: "Exercise, of which walking is a key part."

Dr. Thomas K. Cureton, professor emeritus, Uni-

versity of Illinois, and Director of the Physical Fitness
Institute at the university, is probably the leading ex-
ponent of aerobic conditioning in this country. At the
university they call him Mr. Fitness. Cureton has written 54 books and over 500 articles on fitness. He has
also trained many fitness leaders (580 holders of masters degrees and doctorates in exercise physiology). At
the age of 76, Cureton walks five miles each day. He
does the four-mile round trip to and from his office at
the university—no matter what the weather—and gets
in another mile at noon. If he can't squeeze in 30 minutes after lunch or dinner, he walks before going to
bed. He even makes sure he walks when on a business
trip or vacation. Cureton feels that walking is the best
kind of fitness activity. The all-out, intense effort you
get from many activities such as sports doesn't provide maximum cardiovascular benefits and a maximum reduction in stress. Walking does. The key, according to Cureton, is moderate exercise sustained
over a long period of time. And walking fills that bill
for Cureton. Apparently his ideas work. In 1978, he
won the National Masters Cross Country Champion-
ship for 70-year-olds. He also has several gold medals
from the Masters Track and Field competition.

Dr. Roy Shephard, M.D., Professor, Department of
Physiological Hygiene, the University of Toronto, has
a unique way of building walking into his commuting.
Shephard's home is a 20-minute walk from the bus that
takes him to the university. Each morning he leaves
the home a few minutes later than he should. He must
walk briskly to the bus station to stay on schedule. He
has to walk so fast that his heart rate reaches target
rate levels. This approach gives him a few extra winks,
more time at the breakfast table, and fitness.

Some people, who must drive or travel by public
transportation for several miles to get to work each
day, assume that they cannot walk to work. They can't
walk the entire distance, that's true. But they can do
what Klumpp does: they can park their cars or get off

the train a couple of miles from work and walk the rest of the way.

If you drive to work, you might even save money if you walk part of the way. As every long-distance commuter knows, the longest part of the drive to work is inevitably the last mile or two, as you near the congested area that everyone is trying to reach. If you're really unlucky, it can take the last 10 minutes of an hour-long drive to go just four blocks. If you parked your car four, six, or eight blocks from work, you could probably walk that distance in the same amount of time it takes you to drive, fight for a parking space, and get to your office. And chances are that you'll pay less for parking because you won't be fighting for a prime parking space. Depending on the location, if you play your cards right, you may even be able to find a free space.

Employers could make an important contribution to their employees' welfare and productivity by encouraging them through financial and physical incentives to walk to work. Here is one idea that deserves consideration. A company could rent parking lots a mile or two away from its offices so employees could park there and walk to work. In case of bad weather, umbrellas and perhaps even other rain gear could be placed at the office and parking lots for use by walking employees. This system has the built-in potential for progress checks and awards. Some sort of sign-in and sign-out procedure could be used to check whether employees use the facility. Many companies are already awarding their physically fit employees with special financial incentives. This system would lend itself perfectly to such a program. It could also help companies that don't have facilities for exercise.

The chief financial officer of several companies will read this and think, "Terrific. But how much is all this walking going to cost and who's going to pay for it?" In a way, it would be just like any other investment. It might cost a few dollars at first, but that money would quickly pay dividends in terms of healthier, more productive employees who take fewer days off for illness. And it probably wouldn't hurt a company's insurance rates.

But if this seems too complicated, there are plenty of simple ideas, too. Here's one that wouldn't take more than an hour or two to put into practice. A company could measure the distance from some of the more common subway stations and bus stops to its central office. Suggested times and distances could be recorded. Ford Motor Company in Dearborn, Michigan, has already done this. The company has devised an activity called "The Headquarters Hustle." The Hustle is to encourage employees to exercise during the course of the working day.

To do "The Headquarters Hustle" an employee first visits the Health Services Department and picks up a map of the measured distances throughout the company area. The next step is to chart a daily walking course.

Guidelines included with the map explain that walking can produce cardiovascular fitness if the pace is sufficient and if the exercise is performed three to four times a week. In the guidelines is a starter program for those who are "out of shape."

Dr. Beverly Ware, Corporate Health Education Programs Coordinator at Ford, explains the rationale for the walking program. "We wanted [the employees] to know that they could indeed do something constructive in their working clothes and in a relatively short time period right at the work site, despite not having physical facilities for an exercise program on location."

Urban planners could also help the walker-traveler-commuter. Over a decade ago, Charles Abrams said in his excellent book, *The Cities The Frontier*:

Urbanization in America has reduced the scenes and enticements that encourage walking.

Peripatetic is a waning breed. Even the word "pedestrian" has become an ugly adjective describing the dull, common place and unimaginative, while the word streetwalker now describes a less honorable exercise. Sidewalks are now being narrowed and trees cut down to make room for more cars, and the residue is being cluttered with driveways, vault openings, ash cans, traffic signs, pumps, parking meters, mail boxes—in fact everything but trees and benches.

Abrams recommends that some courageous mayor should appoint a commissioner of pedestrians. This commissioner would protect walkers' rights and maybe even change a few downtown streets into no-car streets, create walkways to public transportation facilities, and build pedestrian "islands."

Two More Walking Commuters

Here are two more examples of how you can walk to work and to fitness at the same time.

Fred Sanders, an acquaintance of Charles T. Kuntzleman, did not like the idea of attending fitness classes. He wouldn't budge. "Nobody's going to get me into an exercise class so I can grunt and groan and hop up and down like a lunatic," he said.

As time went by, however, his extra fat really began to get to him. One day he went to Kuntzleman's exercise class and said, "I want to lose a few pounds and my diet's not working. Maybe I'll give this a try. But I don't want to go to any of those classes, and I don't want to do any exercises."

It was easy to see that Sanders would never stick to a program that required him to do anything but the bare minimum. Sports were out, since he didn't play any and didn't want to learn. He disliked calisthenics, and group activity left him cold. Walking seemed to be more his style; it was less like work.

Sanders was in the habit of driving to the office, even though his area had a good commuter service. Kuntzleman suggested that he leave the car in the garage and take the train into town. "But if I leave the car in the garage, how am I going to get to the station?" he whined. "Walk," Kuntzleman told him, and added, "A half hour at a good brisk clip will burn about 250 calories. You get home again the same way. You also walk half an hour at lunch time—pick a restaurant that's 15 minutes away from your office."

Sanders grumpily agreed. All that walking was not to his liking, but he had to admit it didn't sound too inconvenient. At most, he had to get up a half hour earlier in the morning and arrive home a half hour later in the evening. (He soon found out it was more like 15 minutes.) If he was going to become active, this seemed like the easiest way to go about it.

To his great surprise, once Sanders got into the swing of it, he found he actually enjoyed his walks. He watched the seasons change, something he had never really seen before. He got to know people along his route, but mostly he liked being alone with his thoughts. Frequently, he would let his mind take off on its own and found that solutions to knotty problems came to him—"out of the blue, just like that!"—during his walks.

He slacked off somewhat over the first four months, so all in all, he lost "only" 30 pounds that year. But Sanders is still walking—and losing. Or is it winning?

A woman we'll call Connie is a 43-year-old executive in a brokerage firm. She told Kuntzleman of her interest in walking for fitness. But she had very little free time. Here is the program that Kuntzleman outlined for her.

1. 8:50 A.M. Instead of having the bus let you off in front of the office door, get off five to eight

blocks from the office, and walk at a brisk pace for 10 minutes.

2. 9:00 A.M. A climb up five flights of stairs to your office on the 10th floor. (Connie got off the elevator on the fifth floor and walked the rest of the way up.)

3. Mid-morning. For 10 minutes, walk back and forth in the hall when everyone else is taking a coffee break. (Sometimes to provide a cover for this strange habit, Connie would deliberately schedule a 10-minute errand, or she would go down several flights of stairs to make a call.)

4. Before lunch. Walk down five flights of stairs.

5. Lunchtime. A brisk 15-minute walk to the restaurant; another brisk 15-minute walk back to the office building; walk up five flights of stairs to the 10th floor.

6. Mid-afternoon. Another 10 minutes of walking back and forth in the hall or running another errand.

7. End of the day. Another walk down five flights of stairs; another 10-minute walk at a fast pace before catching the bus.

Did all of this make any difference? Yes. Here are how many calories Connie burned in one day: two 10-minute walks, 133 calories; two 15-minute walks, 200 calories; two walks up five flights of stairs, 25 calories; two walks down five flights of stairs, 25 calories; two 10-minute walking sessions, morning and afternoon, 100 calories. The daily total is 483 calories. Multiply that by five days a week, and you'll see that she had burned 2,415 extra calories each week.

WALK, WEATHER OR NOT

YOU CAN KEEP ON WALKING IN ALL BUT THE WORST KINDS OF WEATHER.

Some days, the weather is going to be ideal for walking: very light breeze, temperature around 60 degrees, no clouds in sight. But what do you do when the snow starts to fall, a gale threatens to blow you off the path, or the heat makes you feel as though your shoes will melt? It may not sound very appealing to you now, but you can walk in all but the very worst weather conditions. If you succeed in making your walking program as much a part of your day as eating or sleeping, you'll probably find yourself walking through rain, snow, and sleet—and enjoying every minute of it.

Temperature extremes can be more than uncomfortable; they can be dangerous if you do not prepare yourself adequately.

Cold weather shouldn't present any serious problems if you are in reasonably good condition. It is just a matter of attitude. If you have heart problems, however, ask your doctor if it is all right for you to brave very cold weather—even if he has already given you permission to walk. High wind-chill factors are the greatest threat in cold weather, since you can get frostbite if you are inadequately protected from the wind. When you walk, your own motion against the wind increases the wind-chill factor and the risk of frostbite. Be sure that all normally exposed areas of your skin—

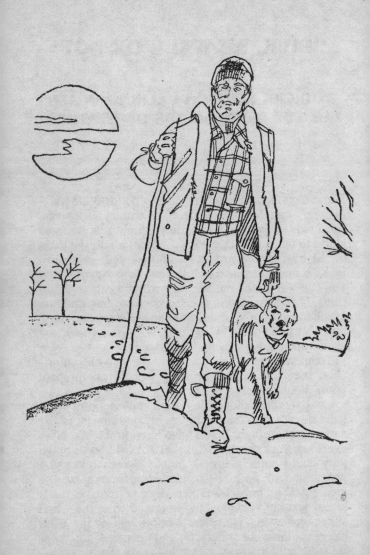

head, face, ears, and hands—are covered. If you are wearing proper clothing, only the bitterest cold should bother you.

When it is hot, be especially careful. Cut down on your usual program. In some instances you may simply have to stop. When the thermometer hits 90 degrees be cautious. Dr. Terry Kavanagh, the doctor who has trained heart attack victims to run marathons, tells his heart patient joggers to quit if it gets warmer than 85 degrees. You are going to have to experiment. But as a rule of thumb, if you are just starting to walk, have heart problems, are overweight, or more than 40 years old, set 85 degrees as your limit.

The real problem with hot weather is humidity. When your body starts to heat up, your body's cooling system is automatically turned on and you begin to sweat. The function of sweating is to keep your body cool. As your blood circulates through you, it heats up at the center part of your body. When the blood comes near the surface of the skin, the sweating and the evaporation of sweat allow the blood to cool. Consequently, your blood temperature drops a bit and the cool blood is circulated back to the center of the body. At the center, the blood heats up again and goes back to the skin. This is how your body maintains the proper temperature in a hot environment. But when the humidity is high, your thermostat doesn't work properly. The sweat doesn't evaporate, and your body temperature continues to rise.

If you continue walking vigorously while sweating profusely, you may run out of water. When this supply of body water is gone, your blood circulation is reduced and your blood pressure falls. The result can be heat exhaustion. Weakness, fainting, and shock may occur. You can avoid heat exhaustion by drinking water before, during, and after the walk. But if you don't drink water, your body temperature will continue to rise and you can get heat stroke. A person who gets heat stroke must be treated immediately. The victim must be placed in a tub of cold water or in a cold shower. If the person's temperature reaches 108 degrees, he will die.

You can avoid heat stroke and heat exhaustion or dehydration by drinking plenty of fluids, wearing light clothing, and, if it is too hot and humid, by backing off. Follow this rule: Drink a full glass of water before you begin, and more during your walk, especially if it lasts more than 30 minutes. You might also try wearing a fishnet vest (or a meshlike fabric) which will help by creating an insulating layer next to your body and thus reducing the temperature.

The only protection between you and the elements when walking is your clothing. A little bit of knowledge on how to select your clothing will go a long way in helping you "weather the weather."

In hot, humid weather, wear something that will let your body breathe as much as possible. Wear as little as you can. For the lower part of the body, nylon underwear is probably the most comfortable you can wear. Cotton is all right, too, but it can cause chafing, partly because it absorbs more perspiration than nylon and partly because the thicker cotton seams tend to irritate the thighs.

Cotton is the best material for the upper body in hot weather. It absorbs perspiration and lets perspiration evaporate easily as you walk. The motto in warm, humid weather is: Lighter is better.

Of course, there is no shortage of expensive fashions. Many walkers wear jogging outfits. These are available in different materials and designs. But if you go this route, don't wear a rubberized, plastic, or otherwise nonporous sweatsuit. In warm or hot weather, you don't want heat and moisture to be trapped. You want it to circulate and escape to keep your body cool. Those who imagine they are undergoing a kind of "Turkish bath" on the hoof are deluding themselves. They may perspire more than someone walking in shorts and lose more water and weight while they walk, but they will promptly regain that lost weight when they rush to the water fountain. The problem is that these clothes create a hot, humid environment and can trigger the phenomena of dehydration, heat exhaustion, and heat stroke. If you want to wear a suit, get one that is porous. It should be made of either cotton or a combination of cotton and a porous synthetic fiber. It should fit loosely without getting in your way.

Body heat is lost through the head, but it is also gained through the head. The head is the first part of the body struck by the powerful rays of the summer sun. So if you protect your head, you can help control your body temperature when you walk in the summer. For this, some walkers prefer to wear a lightweight cap, preferably one that is light colored, to reflect the sun's rays. They feel it keeps the head and the whole body cool.

All of this takes care of walking in Atlanta in July. But what about Central Park in February?

In cold weather, reverse the hot-weather strategy. You need to construct a personal heating system that uses your body as the furnace. To do that, dress in layers of clothing. This is very much like the insulation in your home: it keeps the heat in and the cold out. The layers of clothing trap warm air and hold it next to your body. The more you work, the warmer the air becomes. At the same time, these layers of warm air act as a barrier to the cold. A nylon windbreaker creates the strongest insulation.

After a little practice you will learn quickly what you will need for protection from the cold and the wind. In cold weather, it is always better to be overdressed than underdressed when you walk. That way you can take off clothes if you need to. This extra clothing usually is just a jacket and pants that can be tied around your waist.

In wet weather, leather shoes are better than nylon. That way your feet will stay drier. In very wet weather, put plastic bags over your socks. That may seem absurd, but people have walked in snow with suede shoes for over 10 hours and never had wet socks.

Wear socks when walking. Socks should be made of either cotton or wool. They absorb moisture well. Some walkers prefer cotton over wool because wool can be irritating. This is an individual matter.

Some people like to wear two pairs of socks, especially in cold weather. That's fine as long as one pair is lighter than the other. Don't select nylon as the lighter sock. Nylon socks tend to cause blisters.

There are two basic lengths: anklets that reach just above the shoe top, and socks that go halfway up the calf. Anklets are better for summer walking since they are cool; the calf-high variety is more suited for winter walking because it offers greater protection.

On long walks, men can suffer irritation from athletic supporters, a problem which some walkers have solved with an apparently satisfactory, if unusual, substitute—women's panties. Some manufacturers of shorts have more or less followed the lead by designing "unisex" shorts, worn by men and women alike. Designed with a built-in nylon support, they will not rub, bind, or chafe. Another suggestion is: if you are bothered, don't wear any underwear at all. This may take a little time to get used to, but you may find it best for comfort. Also, a little petroleum jelly on the upper thighs can put an end to chafing.

It has been estimated that a hat or cap holds in 80 percent of the body's heat during winter. Put a cap on your head and, in effect, you've "capped" the heat's escape route. In fact, one walker has said, "If you want to keep your feet warm, wear a hat."

Wear a heavy knitted wool or Orlon ski cap, one you can pull down over your ears and face, when you walk in the winter. This design gives you flexibility. It can protect you from the cold and be conveniently rolled up to form a cap if you don't want to cover your face.

Many people feel the pull-down mask is the only

way to go. When the wind is at your back, you can roll it up and expose your face to the sun's warm rays. But when you are heading into a strong wind, it's handy to pull down over your face to protect it from frostbite.

But a mask is a mixed blessing. Perspiration and condensation of the breath can freeze into ice around your mouth and nostrils—not the most pleasant winter experience. Some walkers have complained that a mask tends to congest the sinuses because it inhibits breathing. Nevertheless, for safety's sake, use a ski mask when the wind-chill factor is high.

Another type of mask is designed to filter polluted air that many people in urban areas must breathe. If you habitually find yourself walking alongside cars and trucks that spew out carbon monoxide, a mask of this type might be worth using.

Mittens, not gloves, give your hands the best protection in cold weather. Mittens don't have separate fingers, so cold air cannot circulate around each one. The fingers and the palm are crowded together, nice and warm in the same air space. Some people use tube socks as mittens because they go well up the arm. In really cold weather some walkers wear mittens with socks on top. Others wear gloves with mittens on top.

Specific Problems

Rain, snow, ice, hail, lightning, strong winds, fog and other harsh weather conditions can curtail your walking. So can high altitudes and darkness. But with a little bit of ingenuity, all of these can be overcome.

On warm days—any temperature higher than 70 degrees—rain is no problem for walkers. You may even welcome it. On days when the temperature dips below 60 degrees, a light rain jacket will give you sufficient protection. If you worry about your hair, you can either buy a special rain hat or carry an umbrella.

Some people love to walk in the snow. To cope with the snow, simply follow the directions for walking in the cold. Your pace will be slower, but that's okay. If the snow is deep, you'll be working just as hard as you would be at a faster pace on a clean street. If you doubt it, check your pulse.

Walking on the ice can be treacherous. It is easy to slip and injure yourself. If there is ice on the road or sidewalk, it is best to wait until later in the day when cars and people have chewed it up or the sun has melted it. If you can't do that, try to find a clean path. If that is impossible, you may walk inside on that day.

Hail can be a problem. If the hail's large, take shelter immediately. If it's small, be your own judge. Most of the time it won't harm you.

At the first sign of any lightning, head for cover. A car or building is best. If you are caught where you can't get to such cover, stay away from water, metal objects, and single trees. The best bet is to get into a hollow or a ditch. Or you might even try hiding under a small bush. Don't take chances. Get down on your knees and bend over as far as possible . . . and pray. Lightning can be deadly.

If you walk in a strong wind, you will be using up more oxygen than you would under ordinary conditions. So, if you're walking into a stiff breeze, you may want to slow down. It's like walking through deep snow. You'll get the same benefits that you would in a faster walk under normal conditions. When you set out to walk on a windy day, start walking into the wind. Then toward the end, when you are perspiring and tired, you'll have the wind to your back. It will not only make your walk easier, but it will help reduce the possibility of getting chilled.

High altitudes are a source of special problems. At 5,000 feet above sea level and higher, there is significantly less oxygen than there is at lower levels, so there is less for your body to absorb. As a result, your heart has to work hard. For every 2,500 feet that you go up, plan on taking at least a week to adjust. One way that you might adjust is to cut your program by 50 percent at the beginning. If you find yourself short of breath even at that rate, slow down even more.

When walking at night, follow these basic guidelines:

1. Face the traffic as you walk, and stay close to the edge of the road. If a car seems to be bearing down on you, step off the road and stop walking.
2. Wear light-colored clothes. White is best. If you want, wear some reflective type of tape, too.
3. Carry a flashlight so that you can see where you are walking and so you can also alert motorists.
4. Know the road you are walking on. That way you'll know where the curves and ditches are.
5. Don't look directly at the headlights of oncoming cars. They tend to blind you, and as a result you can't see where you are going. Look off to the side. You'll still be able to see the car.

Walking in the fog is similar to walking in darkness. Follow all the guidelines for walking in darkness with one exception. Don't wear white, light-colored clothes, especially gray. Bright red or orange clothing is best.

Staying Inside

Walking indoors is a solution to the problems of bad weather conditions. It has drawbacks. There are no bumps, potholes, or cars to worry about; yet walking indoors, going around and around the same track, can be boring. If you are trying to walk a mile, it may take you 20 or more laps to make it. Your mind tends to grow numb, and it is easy to become discouraged.

If you are going to walk on an indoor track for several days or more, it is best to switch direction every other day. By walking counterclockwise one day and clockwise the next, you will help avoid orthopedic problems that can result from walking on a surface that slopes to the left or right.

You can also use an indoor treadmill. A treadmill is nothing more than a conveyer belt for walking. There are two kinds—motorized and nonmotorized.

Walking on a motorized treadmill is as close to real walking as you can get without actually hitting the street. You simulate the walk almost exactly. Many motorized treadmills can be raised at one end to imitate walking uphill, making the exercise more difficult and increasing its value. Most motorized treadmills cost over $1,000.

Nonmotorized treadmills are comparatively inexpensive. They range in price from $150 to $600. They are driven by your own muscle power. They can be uncomfortable and difficult to work for long periods—15 minutes or more. The belt is on rollers, and after a period of walking, people seem to experience a "hot foot" because of the friction. Another problem is that the incline of the treadmill—5 to 10 percent—seems to aggravate leg pain in certain people. The nonmotorized treadmill is fine for slow walking for brief periods of time, but it seems to lead to foot and leg irritation at a fast pace.

SOME SPECIAL SITUATIONS

EVEN PEOPLE WITH SIGNIFICANT HEALTH PROBLEMS CAN USE OUR PROGRAM.

If you've read this far and still haven't decided to begin a walking program following the guidelines we've set up, it could be because you're concerned about some special problems.

In the past, people who'd had heart attacks, suffered from emphysema or arthritis, or were extraordinarily overweight were given medicine or put on diets and were told to take it easy. Today the situation is different. Doctors are now telling their patients to get some exercise. In particular, they are telling them to walk.

As we've said before, if you have questions about your health or are seeing a doctor regularly for specific problems, do not begin a walking program until you have received permission and specific instructions from your doctor. We think you should go ahead and ask about walking, no matter how serious your condition. Chances are, your doctor will allow you to begin, even if you have one of the special problems discussed below.

Obesity

This is a serious problem throughout the developed (overdeveloped?) world. Between 20 and 50 percent of

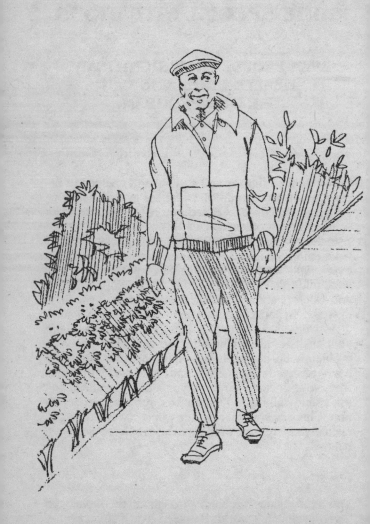

all Americans have too much fat. Recent studies in Canada indicate that as much as 75 percent of all Canadians worry about their present weight. Americans worry too. Obesity—being grossly, not just a few pounds, overweight—has become an increasing health problem in recent years. Many doctors and experts on obesity have felt that obese people either will not or should not exercise. But the phenomenal success of many obese people in walking programs has prompted some new thinking. Obese people probably will not lose weight through extremely strenuous physical activity; yet they can achieve excellent results through walking.

Let's examine some of the causes of obesity and the reasons why walking has been a successful means of helping obese people to lose weight.

Hunger is perhaps one of the most misunderstood words in our vocabulary. It refers to the craving for food that is usually associated with a number of unpleasant sensations. A person who has had no food for many hours will have stomach contractions, often called hunger pangs. This is the gnawing sensation that you experience at 11 in the morning if you skipped breakfast. Most of us, fortunately, have never known the severe pain of acute hunger suffered by millions of starving people around the world. Therefore, most of us do not understand true hunger.

Appetite is often confused with hunger. Appetite is the desire for a specific type of food, such as strawberries, milk, pizza, cookies. Your appetite determines the kind of food you eat.

Satiety means complete fulfillment—the absence of both hunger and appetite—even though food may be available.

The stomach does not control hunger. Even a person who has had part or all of his stomach removed will continue to feel hungry. Hunger is a response of the hypothalamus, a tiny part of the brain, to the fluctuating glucose level of the blood: the "glucostatic regulation of food intake."

In simple terms, according to the "glucostatic theory," when the blood glucose concentration falls too far, the part of the hypothalamus that signals satiety reduces its inhibiting effects on the part that controls the hunger sensation. An impulse is sent from the hypothalamus to the stomach. When the stomach gets the signal, stomach contractions begin. This causes the feeling of hunger. Although there are still missing links in this theory, there is more scientific evidence to support it than any other concept.

It is not known what determines either the size of the meal eaten or the sense of fullness after a meal. Scientists think that there are receptors of some type in the gastrointestinal tract that may trigger a nervous or hormonal mechanism, which in turn activates the hypothalamic satiety center. This process may be triggered by taste and smell, the number of fat deposits in the body, amino acid imbalance, glucose released by the liver, and glucagon (a protein that elevates blood glucose levels).

Calories (found only in proteins, fats, and carbohydrates) are essential, therefore, to satisfy hunger for any period of time. Bulk has very little to do with satisfying hunger. The sense of fullness that many people experience when they eat low-calorie or noncaloric foods may be caused by receptors in the gastrointestinal tract, but the feeling of fullness does not last long. This prompts the old saying that certain foods don't "stick to your ribs."

This is a serious indictment of noncaloric foods. People who use diet sodas, soups, crackers, cookies, etc., in an effort to reduce weight are just kidding themselves. They may lose weight at first, but their hunger will continue because of low glucose levels. As a result they will be continually hungry.

In one experiment, rats were given a certain amount of food over a period of time. Activity and diet were maintained at a constant level, and the rats were able to hold a steady weight. The researchers then changed 10 percent of the diet to noncaloric food that was very similar to diet foods used by people. When the new food contained 10 percent inert material (no calories), the rats ate approximately 10 percent more food. When the researchers raised the noncaloric portion to 20 percent, the animals ate 20 percent more food. This trend continued as the proportion of noncaloric food was increased. Finally, the animals literally ate themselves to death attempting to satisfy their appetites with low-calorie, high-bulk foods.

The glucostatic theory explains why some foods satisfy hunger and others don't. It is still not clear why some people crave more food than others and seem to be hungry all the time, but there are several theories.

The Appestat Theory. Scientists call the feeding and satiety center of the hypothalamus the appestat. It is the regulator that controls appetite. This regulator seems to be set a little higher in some people than in others. The person whose appestat is set higher usually has greater difficulty in controlling weight. Although experiencing both hunger and satiety, the person with a high setting needs a little more food (glucose, to which all proteins, carbohydrates, or fats are eventually converted) to satisfy the satiety center, or appestat. Exactly why the appestat is sometimes set too high is not clear. Many scientists nevertheless feel that this theory provides perhaps one of the more logical explanations of why people gain weight.

In primitive cultures, human beings had to be physically active to survive. A high appestat setting was an advantage: a person with a higher setting experienced greater hunger and pursued food much more aggressively than a person with a lower setting. As a result, that person hunted down, ate, and stored more food so that his or her body had additional energy at hand and more body tissue. During periods when little or no food could be found, stored body fat and tissue provided sustenance until food was found. The person with the lower appestat setting had less stored energy and body tissue. (Of course, the person who remained physically active in the pursuit and preparation of food never became obese.)

In modern Western society, the situation is reversed. Vigorous physical activity is no longer required to obtain and prepare food, but we still have appestats. Nowadays, if you have a high appestat setting, you are at a disadvantage. The evolutionary instinct to eat more food so that you will be able to survive in a period of crisis continues to operate, but today you are likely to be underexercised. You don't burn up the excess calories, so you gain weight. And, unless you become marooned on a desert island, chances are slim that a nutritional crisis will occur in your lifetime. So the pounds continue to add up.

You can, of course, restrict your caloric intake, but you will experience a continual hunger, a hunger that is constantly stimulated by food ads on TV, billboards, magazines, and newspapers. Your appestat will demand that the hunger be satisfied. Since hunger is satisfied by increasing caloric intake, unless you are extremely strong-willed, practically any diet is doomed to failure.

The Psychological Theory. According to this theory, obesity and overweight are by-products of psychological problems or of conditioning. A researcher can cause a rat to overeat by punishing it if it does not. This kind of conditioning occurs in human beings, too. Many children eat and overeat in an effort to win their parents' approval, or in some cases, to avoid punishment. Some well-meaning parents still believe that "a fat child is a healthy child" and expect their children to overeat. Also, some parents and other adults give children cookies or candy as a reward for good behavior, or to distract them from crying after a fall.

A child's first exposure to overeating often occurs very early in life. Dr. Hilde Bruch, professor of psychiatry at Baylor College of Medicine, states that a baby's tears are often misinterpreted as hunger. Unfortunately, many adults thrust a bottle in the mouth of a crying infant instead of considering whether the need may be for cuddling, comfort, a change of diaper, or a change of scene. Therefore, it's only natural that the child learns to link emotional and physical needs with eating. If food is used to placate needs other than hunger, a child may be conditioned to want food even when not hungry.

Another aspect of the psychological theory focuses on the role of tension and frustration in overeating. Stress situations (death of a parent, loss of a job, etc.) can cause you to eat nervously if you were so conditioned in childhood, and also to refrain from physical activity. In fact, you may want to sleep more, or you may become depressed and just want to sit.

The most interesting aspect of the psychological theory is the observation that obese and overweight people tend to become less active. This compounds the problem. Dr. Albert Stunkard has observed that situations that cause overeating also lead to decreased physical activity and that a person who experiences periods of intense depression may also undergo a significant change in carbohydrate metabolism.

Obesity and overweight contribute to inactivity, and inactivity begets weight gain. It is indeed a vicious circle. Dr. M. F. Graham, of Dallas, Texas, has illustrated that cycle in a diagram (page 152).

The Graham diagram shows the usual progression: stress, anxiety, and tension lead to compulsive eating, which shows up as fat (obesity and overweight), which leads to physical inactivity, and therefore greater stress, anxiety, and tension. Physical activity is the simplest means of breaking the vicious cycle outlined by Graham.

The appestat and psychological theories are both valid. In many instances, obesity and overweight result from a combination of causes. What you must

FIGURE 1/THE OVEREATING CYCLE

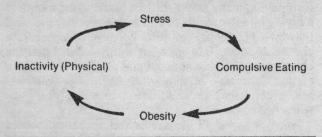

M. F. Graham, *Prescription For Life*. New York: David McKay, 1966, p. 43.

remember is that physical activity is the most reliable way to control weight. Also, when people exercise regularly, they don't look as flabby as most dieters. They like what they see in the mirror. Muscles are taut. Breasts do not sag. Abdomens are flat—almost washboardlike. The body is attractive and desirable.

If you are obese or very much overweight, your goal in walking should be to walk as far as you can. Don't worry about speed; distance is far more important. There are two reasons for this.

At rest, most of our energy comes from carbohydrates stored in the body. In short bursts of effort such as sprinting, practically all our energy comes from glycogen. During such exercises as walking a half hour or so, jogging, or swimming, about 50 percent of our energy comes from glycogen and 50 percent from the fat. If you exercise for an hour, there will be a significant increase in the amount of fat used. And if you exercise even longer than that, fat will supply almost 90 percent of the needed energy. So the longer you go, the most fat you burn.

Physics tells us that it takes just as much energy to move an object slowly as it does to move it quickly. Your body doesn't violate that principle. If you compare walking with jogging at moderate speeds, you will find very little difference between them in terms of energy requirements. In one mile of jogging, the average American will burn about 100 calories; in one mile of walking, he'll burn about 90 to 95 calories. If you run a mile in 10 minutes, you will burn about 10 calories per minute; if you walk a mile in 20 minutes, you will burn about five calories per minute.

If you are obese, you still can exercise, provided you do it in the manner that has been outlined. You must follow this go-slow approach. That is a hard lesson to learn, especially if you are a competitive individual. Don't walk at an unrealistic pace. You'll become exhausted and discouraged. Use distance (or time) and go at a pace you can cope with. Follow the tables in our program and focus on going a minimum of four times a week. If you are extremely obese and find this difficult, you can follow one of the cardiac programs outlined in the next few pages. Your goal should be to work at your target heart rate for a miminum of 30 minutes. When this amount of walking no longer allows you to reach your target heart rate, you can gradually increase to 60 minutes or more of walking a day.

Heart Attack Victims

Heart disease sufferers can benefit from walking. Dr. Albert Kattus, chairman of the Exercise Committee for the American Heart Association and professor of medicine (cardiology) at UCLA, is a strong proponent of walking for people who have heart problems. Several years ago, he and some associates studied 50 people with angina (chest pain). The patients were urged to walk farther and farther each day. At first, 100 feet three times a day was the limit. As their conditioning improved, some eventually walked two miles. A full 75 percent of the patients improved. Five of the patients said that their angina disappeared. Tests showed that where the arteries had been closed off, the heart, by expanding small arteries, had built new "bridges" of circulation around them.

What is exciting about Kattus's study is that these are not isolated examples. Some people have run marathons after suffering heart attacks. They didn't start by running; they started by walking. Doctors now know that something happens to heart disease sufferers who exercise. Dr. Kenneth Cooper describes it this way:

> Aerobic exercise increases the cells of your body. New vessels may appear as if from nowhere—perhaps because the physical stimulus of the vigorous circulation or perhaps by some chemical trigger: we don't know the cause, but the result is that when you get your heart rate up during an aerobic exercise workout, the cells throughout your body get a better cleansing and more life-sustaining oxygen than they did before.

Again, our emphasis is on the practical. Use your doctor's guidelines as limits; that is, how fast and how far. Don't push yourself to the point of pain or to the point of extreme discomfort. If you're excessively tired, or you don't feel right, back off.

TABLE 1. CARDIAC PROGRAM 1

Below is a walking program you can follow if you have had a heart attack and your doctor's approval to exercise. This program assumes that your recovery is normal and uncomplicated. It also implies no necessity for medication for relief of pain and prevention of heart irregularities. Your physician must establish your Target Heart Rate. This will be done via a stress test. The test will indicate how high your heart rate may safely go.

Level 1	3 to 5 minutes	3 times a week
Level 2	6 to 8 minutes	3 times a week
Level 3	9 to 11 minutes	3 times a week

Level 4	12 to 14 minutes	4 times a week
Level 5	15 to 17 minutes	4 times a week
Level 6	18 to 20 minutes	4 times a week
Level 7	21 to 23 minutes	4 times a week
Level 8	24 to 26 minutes	4 times a week
Level 9	27 to 29 minutes	4 times a week
Level 10	30 to 32 minutes	4 times a week
Level 11	33 to 35 minutes	4 times a week
Level 12	36 to 38 minutes	4 times a week
Level 13	39 to 41 minutes	4 times a week
Level 14	42 to 44 minutes	4 times a week
Level 15	45 to 47 minutes	4 times a week
Level 16	48 to 50 minutes	4 times a week
Level 17	51 to 53 minutes	4 times a week
Level 18	54 to 56 minutes	4 times a week
Level 19	57 to 59 minutes	4 times a week
Level 20	60 minutes	4 times a week

TABLE 2. CARDIAC PROGRAM 2

Below is a walking program for those heart attack sufferers who need medication to manage their disease. The walking program should be followed in a medically supervised class. Your physician must establish your Target Heart Rate. This will be done via a stress test. That test will indicate how high your heart rate may safely go.

Level 1:	Walk 1 minute, rest 1 minute, walk 1 minute, rest 1 minute, walk 1 minute, rest 1 minute, walk 1 minute.	3 times a week
Level 2:	Walk 1 minute, rest 1 minute, walk 3 minutes, rest 1 minute, walk 3 minutes, rest 1 minute, walk 1 minute.	3 times a week
Level 3:	Walk 1 minute, rest 1 minute, walk 5 minutes, rest 1 minute, walk 5 minutes, rest 1 minute, walk 1 minute.	3 times a week
Level 4:	Walk 1 minute, rest 1 minute, walk 7 minutes, rest 1 minute, walk 7 minutes, rest 1 minute, walk 1 minute.	3 to 4 times a week

Level 5:	Walk 1 minute, rest 1 minute, walk 8 minutes, rest 1 minute, walk 8 minutes, rest 1 minute, walk 1 minute.	3 to 4 times a week
Level 6:	Walk 1 minute, rest 1 minute, walk 9 minutes, rest 1 minute, walk 9 minutes, rest 1 minute, walk 1 minute.	3 to 4 times a week
Level 7:	Walk 1 minute, rest 1 minute, walk 10 minutes, rest 1 minute, walk 10 minutes, rest 1 minute, walk 1 minute.	3 to 4 times a week
Level 8:	Walk 1 minute, rest 1 minute, walk 11 minutes, rest 1 minute, walk 11 minutes, rest 1 minute, walk 1 minute.	4 times a week
Level 9:	Walk 1 minute, rest 1 minute, walk 12 minutes, rest 1 minute, walk 12 minutes, rest 1 minute, walk 1 minute.	4 times a week
Level 10:	Walk 1 minute, rest 1 minute, walk 14 minutes, rest 1 minute, walk 14 minutes, rest 1 minute, walk 1 minute.	4 times a week
Level 11:	Walk 1 minute, rest 1 minute, walk 16 minutes, rest 1 minute, walk 16 minutes, rest 1 minute, walk 1 minute.	4 times a week
Level 12:	Walk 1 minute, rest 1 minute, walk 18 minutes, rest 1 minute, walk 18 minutes, rest 1 minute, walk 1 minute.	4 times a week
Level 13:	Walk 1 minute, rest 1 minute, walk 20 minutes, rest 1 minute, walk 20 minutes, rest 1 minute, walk 1 minute.	4 times a week

Progress to Level 7 on Cardiac Program #1 when you reach Level 13 on this program.

Arthritis

If you have arthritis, you can walk safely, but like those who are obese and victims of heart disease, you must proceed cautiously. Some people have had arthritis so severe that during the initial stages of their walking program they walked in a pool, because, with the water to keep them buoyant, they weighed less and their joints were subjected to less stress. These were extreme cases, but they illustrate an important principle: don't walk during acute phases of the disease. When the pain is intense, rest.

Sam Poston is the director of Human Services at a small community college. He is a young man, 28, yet he is plagued with arthritic knees. In January 1978, he weighed 213 pounds and had 30 percent body fat. That was when he joined a walking class. At first he only went 20 minutes at a time. Gradually he increased until he was doing three times that much. His weight started to tumble (with help from his diet). Today he weighs 160 pounds, less than he did when he was in eighth grade. Interestingly, he is convinced that the walking has helped his arthritic knees. "I have pain every day, but that is arthritis," he says. "I've never been better, though, because I'm carrying a lot less weight. My leg muscles are a lot stronger to compensate for my knees."

It is impossible to say exactly how much walking you should do. There are too many variables. However, if you have minimal pain, you can probably begin with the Starter Program we've outlined, then progress accordingly. During the first few weeks or months, avoid the target heart rate. If the disease is moderate, you can then try the Cardiac Program 1. If the disease is more severe, you can then try Cardiac Program 2. You must be the judge. You might try walking just to the point of pain. Of course, stay within the guidelines of the chart you select.

Emphysema

According to the United States Public Health Service, 14 million Americans are afflicted with chronic obstructive respiratory disease. By far the most common of these ailments is emphysema. It ranks second only to heart disease as a crippler of men in their most productive years. It causes more invalidism among males than strokes, tuberculosis, and mental disorders combined. But walking can help. It is a good exercise, and possibly the best therapy, for the emphysema sufferer.

Emphysema causes an increase in the size of the alveoli (air cells) in the lungs and the destruction of capillaries. Total lung volume is increased, but the victim's actual breathing capacity is diminished. The progression of the disease is insidious. Sometimes it begins with occasional spells of coughing, and a build-up of phlegm. Unfortunately, this deceptive beginning allows the condition to progress to a more critical stage.

Both absence of activity and overexertion are dangerous for someone with emphysema. A lack of activity will make a person greatly dependent upon others, while overexertion will make breathing very difficult and frightening. As a result, the emphysema sufferer is afraid to do almost anything. He's afraid to move. Every physical effort makes him feel exhausted. So he does less and less. And the less he does, the worse he feels.

Walking is perhaps the simplest of all exercises for the emphysema patient, but it can be frightening at first. At the beginning of a program, a person's hands may turn blue when he walks. It takes a lot of courage to continue.

Yet research shows that if you start slowly, you will be able to make dramatic improvements. Although the walking will not restore lung function, it will improve the circulatory system's capacity. This means that the emphysema patient will be able to do more work. About 10 years ago, Dr. David Christie pursuaded 11 men suffering from emphysema to exercise. The men were to do easy exercises such as arm circling and trunk twisting for 15 minutes. That was followed by slow walk. Some men walked a full mile; others walked only half the distance. The program was keyed individually to the capabilities of each participant. Climbing stairs or bench stepping was also involved in the regimen. That was their daily exercise program.

But it did not stop there. Each man was urged to integrate physical activity into every aspect of his life. "Instead of driving to the corner store, walk," Christie told them. "If you're going to the second floor of the building, walk up the stairs. Don't take the elevator."

There were no miracles. But at the end of two months, nine of the 11 men said that they were able to go through their daily schedules with less difficulty than before. Even the exercising was less tiring than it had been at the start of the program.

The results were far more rewarding than had been expected. Christie had expected the men to develop the psychological ability to tolerate more difficulty in breathing when walking. Predictably, that happened. But to Christie's surprise, he noticed that actual physiological changes also occurred. Maximum exercise levels and duration increased measurably. So did the amount of oxygen the men were able to make use of each minute. There were indications that more oxygen was reaching the blood and that the suffocation associated with emphysema was lessening. Christie speculated that the physiological changes occurred because of new blood vessels in the lungs.

Dr. John Boyer, a San Diego cardiologist and past president of the American College of Sports Medicine, achieved similar results with a group of emphysema patients. He noted that although he could not produce any significant changes with respect to breathing function, the people were able to tolerate greater amounts of exercise (due to better circulation) and that they felt better than before. They felt they could accomplish a great deal more work and they felt less dependent on others.

Because of all this, physicians are recommending exercise as a means of helping emphysema patients. It's not always easy, however. The emphysema patient often feels poorly. But if he can begin walking gradually even if it's only a few feet, he will soon find that by gradually increasing the distance he will be able to comfortably walk for five, 10, 15, and possibly even 30 minutes.

The type of program we suggest for the emphysema patient is the same as Cardiac Program 2. It may take these patients a little longer to go up the chart than it would most people, but that's nothing to worry about. Progress at your own level and pace, stopping when you need to. As you improve, you'll start to feel strong and want to do more and more. Don't worry about speed. Listen to your body.

You won't change the condition of the disease. The damage is done, because of excessive smoking and/or living in a polluted environment. But you can expect your circulation to improve. As the circulation improves, you will be able to accomplish more than you'd imagined you could.

EXERCISES FOR WALKERS

HERE ARE SOME EXCELLENT WAYS TO CONDITION YOUR WHOLE BODY.

The one exercise that will provide complete fitness for all parts of a person's body has not been devised. All exercises have their shortcomings. Swimmers and cyclists, unless they do specific exercises in addition to swimming and cycling, have poor abdominal strength. Yogis lack cardiovascular fitness.

Walking—though good for stamina, weight control and attractive legs—does little for the muscles of the upper body. It will not strengthen your arms, neck, shoulders, and abdomen.

Walking will help you lose weight without tearing down desirable lean body tissue. But it really won't build huge biceps or add inches elsewhere. So, while you may start out looking like a big pear, if you don't exercise your entire body as you move ahead with your walking program, you'll probably end up looking like a smaller pear.

Furthermore, walking will not improve your flexibility in general (although it will enable arthritics to keep their affected joints flexible). A lack of flexibility can set you up for injuries. One complaint often heard from walkers is that before they began their walking program they could touch their toes, but after six months of walking, they can't. The reason is that walking causes the muscles in the back of the legs to contract. Repeated contractions shorten these muscles, tendons and ligaments. To prevent this, you may want to begin doing some stretching exercises.

Therefore, we recommend the following sequence of exercises:

1. Flexibility exercises
2. Calisthenics
3. Walking
4. More calisthenics
5. More flexibility exercises

The following is a list of flexibility exercises and calisthenics. Do you have to do all of them? No. We recommend the first four flexing exercises and two or three of the calisthenics for your warm-up period; the other five flexing exercises and two or three more calisthenics for your cool-down period.

How long should you hold the flexibility exercises, and how many times should you repeat each calisthenic? At first, stretch and hold each flexing move for 10 seconds; gradually build up to 30 seconds. Start out with five repetitions of the selected calisthenics; gradually build up to 30 "reps."

Flexing

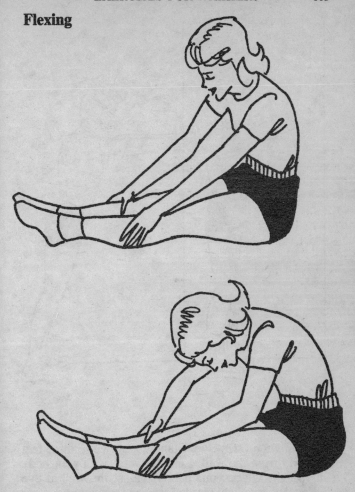

1. **Sitting toe touches.** Sit with your legs extended in front of you on the floor, feet together. Reach for your toes with both hands, and bring your forehead as close to your knees as possible.

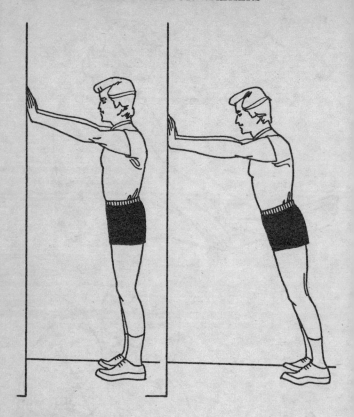

2. **Calf tendon stretches.** Stand about two to three feet
away from the wall. Lean forward, with your body
straight. Place your palms against the wall at eye
level. Step backward. Continue to support your
weight with your hands. Remain flat-footed until
you feel your calf muscles stretching.

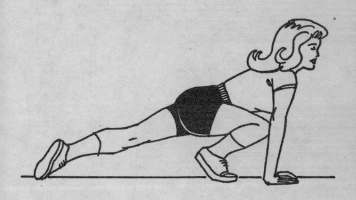

3. **Sprinter.** Assume a squatting position. Then extend one leg backward as far as possible. Your hands should be touching the floor. Hold. Then repeat with the other leg.

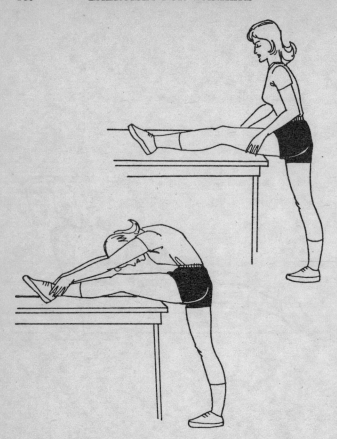

4. **Standing leg stretches.** Find a chair or table approximately three feet in height. Place one foot on the table so that the knee is straight and the leg is parallel to the floor. Slowly extend your fingertips towards the outstretched leg on the table. Eventually you should be able to get your forehead to your knee. Repeat with the other leg.

Calisthenics

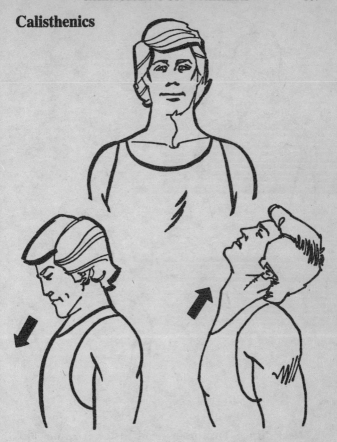

1. **Head flexor.** Assume a standing position with your arms at your sides. Flex your head forward by dropping the chin to your chest. Try to draw your chin down as far as possible. Then extend your head backward as far as possible. This exercise improves neck flexibility and also can help firm muscles in the front of the neck.

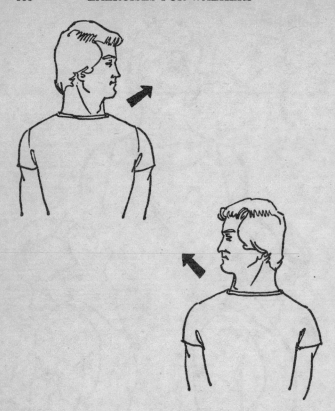

2. **Neck turns.** Turn your head to the left, and look over your left shoulder. Then turn it to the right and look over your right shoulder. This exercise is good for neck flexibility.

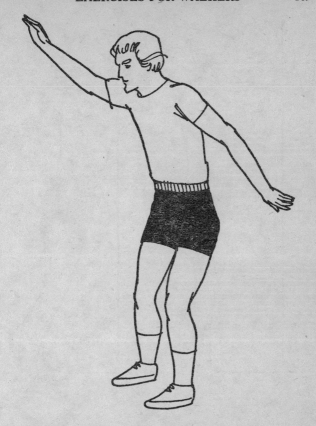

3. **Alternate arm swing and bounce.** Stand with your feet parallel and shoulder-width apart, knees bent at a 45-degree angle. Your body should lean forward, and your arms should hang relaxed. Swing one arm forward as the other one swings back. Continue by reversing the position of your arms with an easy swinging motion. As the motion is continued, bend your knees more than the 45-degree angle and then straighten them. Try to coordinate them. This exercise firms your leg muscles and improves shoulder flexibility.

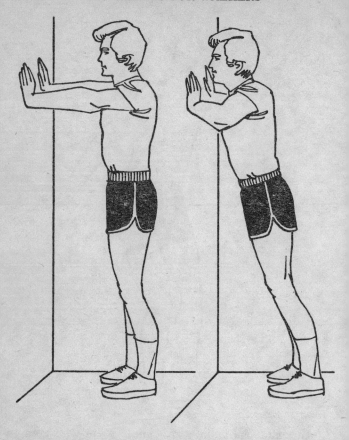

4. **Wall push-up.** Stand about three to four feet away
from the corner or wall of a room. Place one hand
on each wall at shoulder height. Keeping your body
rigid, slowly bend your arms and touch your chin to
the wall or corner. Take three seconds to go into
the wall and three seconds to return. This helps to
strengthen your arm and shoulder muscles.

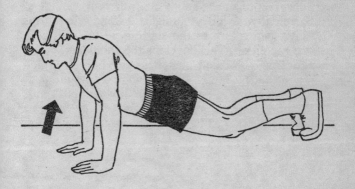

5. **Modified push-up.** Start in a lying position, hands outside the shoulders, fingers pointed forward, and knees bent. Lift your body (from the knees up) off the floor by straightening your arms and keeping your back straight. Return to the starting position. This exercise firms the muscles on the back of your arms.

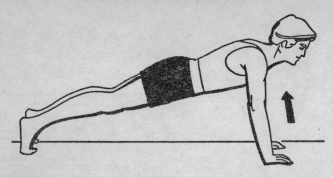

6. **Regular push-up.** Assume a prone position on the floor, feet together, hands beneath your shoulders. Keeping your body straight, extend your arms fully, then return to the starting position. That is one repetition. This develops the shoulders, chest, and arms. Modified push-ups may be substituted for regular push-ups. Women should not automatically substitute modified for regular push-ups. Women can do regular push-ups as well as modified. You just have to understand your limitations.

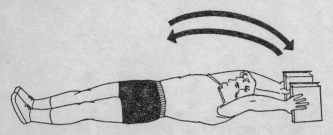

7. **Arms over.** Hold a book in each hand while lying on your back. Extend your arms toward your knees. Then raise the books over your head, reaching as far back as possible. Perform three sets of eight repetitions.

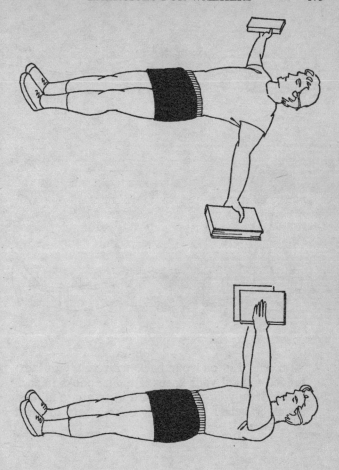

8. **Right angles.** Lie on your back with your arms at
   right angles to your body. Hold a book in each
   hand. Raise your arms so that they point straight
   up, pulling in your abdomen at the same time. Perform three sets of eight repetitions.

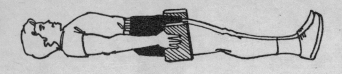

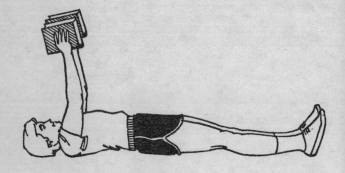

9. **Arm arc.** Lie on your back with your arms extended toward your knees. Holding books in each hand, draw your arms upward in an arc to at least shoulder height. Return. Do three sets of eight repetitions.

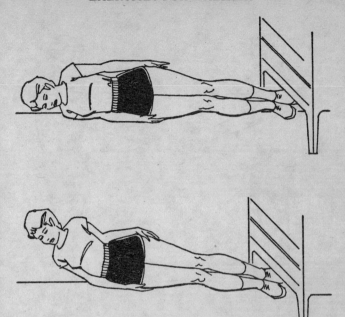

10. **Side bend-up.** Lying on your side with your legs
    held down by a partner or a piece of furniture,
    raise your body sideways from the waist. Raise it
    as high as you can. Do this for both sides.

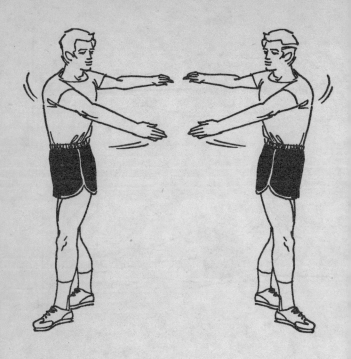

11. **Body twist.** Step forward with your left foot, twist your upper torso to the left as far as possible, and swing both arms to the left. Then step forward with your right foot, twist your upper torso to the right as far as possible, and swing both arms to the right. Exhale as your body twists to the side. Inhale as your body returns to the forward position. This exercise is good for helping stretch abdominal muscles and those in the lower back region.

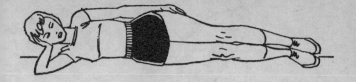

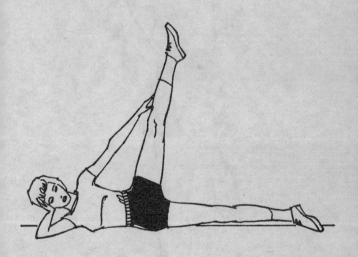

12. **Single leg raise.** Lie on your right side, legs extended, right hand supporting your head. Raise your left leg as high as possible. Lower to the starting position. Start on the right side and then on the left side.

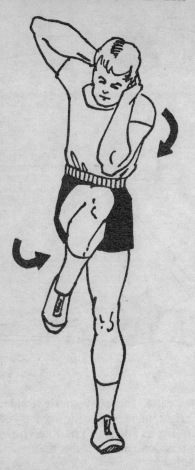

13. **Trunk twister.** Stand with your hands clasped behind your neck and elbows drawn back. As you walk in place, raise your knee as high as possible, and turn the body to the left with your right elbow touching your left knee. Touching of your right elbow to your left knee is one repetition. Repeat for the other side. This exercise conditions your waist and improves your hip flexors.

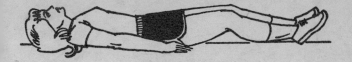

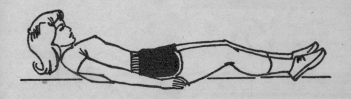

14. **Look-up.** Lie on your back, knees slightly bent and arms at your side. Raise your head and shoulders from the floor until you can see your feet. Lower your head to the floor. The look-up and return is one repetition.

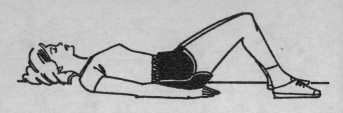

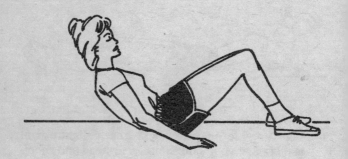

15. **Abdominal curl.** Lie flat on your back with your lower back touching the floor, knees bent. Curl your head and upper part of your body upward and forward to about a 45-degree angle. At the same time, contract your abdominal muscles. Return slowly to the starting position. The curl-up and return is one repetition.

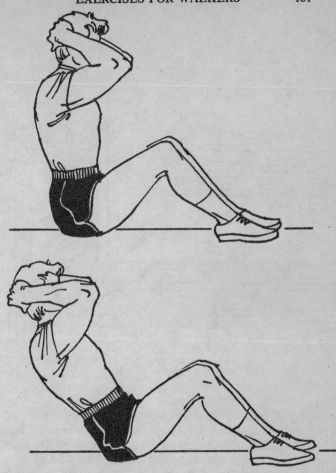

16. **Curl-down.** Start from a sitting position with your knees bent and hands placed behind your head. Lower your upper body to a 45-degree angle. Hold that position and return for one repetition.

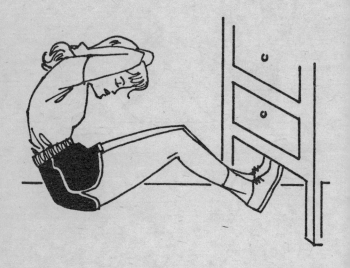

17. **Sit-up.** Lie flat on your back with knees bent and
arms locked behind your head or at your side. You
can brace your feet under a desk or table. Curl
your body into a sitting position by first placing
your chin on your chest and then lifting the upper
part of your body off the floor. Keep your back
rounded. Touch your elbows to your knees. Then
return to the starting position. That is one repetition. You can place your hands above your head
or across your chest if you like.

More Flexing

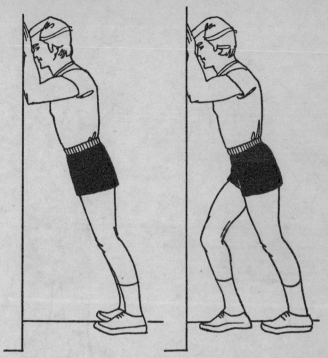

1. **Calf/Achilles stretch.** Face a wall or corner—anything you can lean against. Stand a few feet away from the wall. Rest your forearms on it, and place your forehead on the back of your hands. Bend your right knee, and bring it toward the wall. Keep your left leg straight. Be certain that your left heel remains on the floor. Keep your toes pointed straight ahead. Hold. You should feel the stretching in your calf. Then bend the left knee. Hold. You should feel the stretching in your Achilles tendon. Repeat with your other leg.

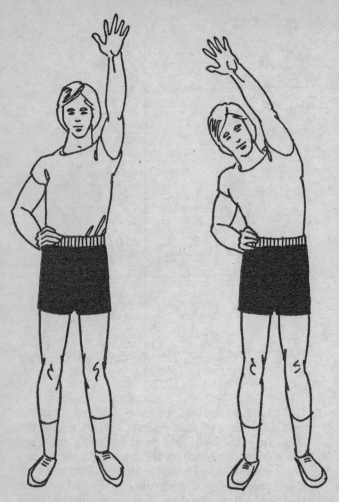

2. **Side stretch.** Stand with your feet about shoulder-width apart. Keep your legs straight. Place one hand on your hip, and extend your other arm up and over your head. Bend to the side on which your hand is placed. Move slowly. Hold. Repeat on the other side.

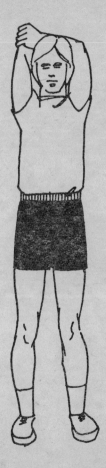

3. **Shoulder stretch.** With your arms over your head,
   hold the elbow of one arm with the hand of the
   other arm. Slowly pull the elbow behind your head.
   Do not force. Hold. Repeat on the other side.

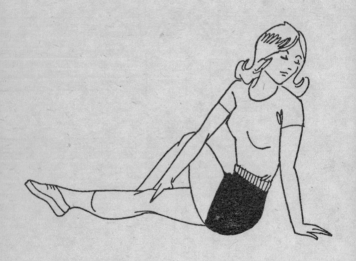

4. **Spinal stretch.** Sit on the floor with your legs straight in front of you. With your right leg straight, put your left foot on the floor on the other side of your right knee. Reach over your left leg with your right arm so that your elbow is on the outside of your left leg. Twist your upper body to the left, and place your right elbow on the outside of your left knee. Hold. Repeat on the other side.

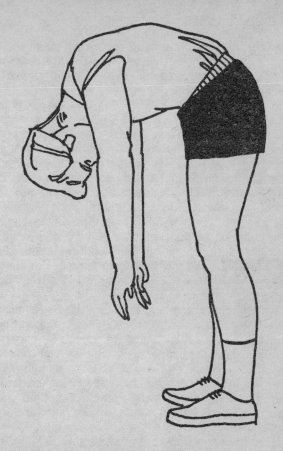

5. **Back stretch.** Stand erect with your feet shoulder-width apart. Bend forward slowly at the waist. Let your arms, shoulders, and neck relax. Go to the point where you feel a slight stretch on the back of your legs. If you cannot go to the floor, place your hands on the backs of your legs. That will give you support. Hold. Remember, when you come back up, bend your knees to take the pressure off your lower back.

Walking Faster

Between these warm-up and cool-down exercises, of course, you will be walking. And there are several things you will want to keep in mind as you get started and as you improve.

What many people call "getting into shape" is just another way of stating a well-known physiological principle: your body adapts to the stress placed on it. And if you want to improve physically, you must put stress on your body over and over again. You must "overload" your body. Dr. Theodore Klumpp, medical consultant for the President's Council on Physical Fitness and Sports, says, "You must push yourself to the point of breathlessness, regardless of your age." The point of breathlessness will vary considerably from person to person, but don't confuse it with gasping. Breathlessness means deep breathing. You should still be able to hold a conversation with someone next to you.

To get to the point of breathlessness you should walk faster and farther. For most people, faster is better than farther because it saves time. You may find that it is the most economical thing for you too. But don't ever forget: how fast you go depends upon your current physical condition. Don't get locked into a chart that tells you to walk a mile at a certain pace. That can be dangerous. You and your pulse are your best guides.

Here is one example of what we mean. Mary is a young woman (37) who lives in Jackson, Michigan. She is very unfit and weighs almost 250 pounds. After five minutes of walking, her pulse is over 85 percent of her predicted maximum heart rate. She is breathing hard, almost wheezing, yet her pace is only two miles per hour. Mary must stop and rest or slow down before going on for another five minutes. If Mary were forced to follow a chart that says she must walk one mile in 15 minutes or less, she would be in serious trouble and probably would give up.

Her feelings of breathlessness, fatigue, and target heart rate are her best guide, not some artificial charts made for some mythical man and woman. You must learn to go at your own pace. It's quite simple: walk faster when your original pace no longer seems to be a challenge.

Do you need more than just walking to accomplish your fitness goals? We can't answer that question for you. You may find that walking all by itself is sufficient to make you feel better than you ever did before you began walking regularly. Then again, you may find your body craving some of these flexing exercises and calisthenics, perhaps even walking in competition. It's likely that your increased awareness of your body that comes as a result of regular brisk walking will stimulate you to pursue other forms of physical conditioning. That's excellent—provided, of course, that you do not cause yourself pain or other discomfort.

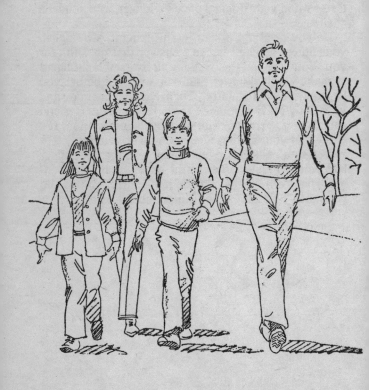

FUTURE GENERATIONS

ENCOURAGE YOUR KIDS: MAKE WALKING A FAMILY AFFAIR.

When you first saw the title of this chapter, you might have said to yourself, "We don't have to worry about the kids—they get lots of exercise." They probably do get more exercise than you, and seem very active . . . perhaps aggravatingly so.

But consider these questions:

How much time do your children (or grandchildren) spend watching television rather than riding their bikes or playing tag? Your children may participate in sports at school, but are these activities truly aerobic? Do your children walk to school, or do you drive them to their classes?

You're certainly not doing it purposely, to be sure, but you're probably bringing up your children to lead sedentary lives. Your children have been mimicking your behavior. Studies prove this to be true.

About 10 years ago, William A. Ruffer completed a study while at the University of Michigan that showed that children's attitudes toward exercise and activity reflect their parents' positions—literally and figuratively. Active high-school students had active parents who encouraged their children to be active; inactive children had inactive parents who did not encourage activity.

That point was driven home to Charles T. Kuntzleman several years ago.

I've exercised regularly since 13 years of age. It's a part of my life. I walk, jog, swim, bicycle, lift weights, and do calisthenics. One day after a run I came in the house and started to do my calisthenics. Two of my children were in the room playing with their friends. The two playmates suddenly stopped playing and turned around and watched in awe. They immediately asked, "What is your dad doing? Why is he doing that?" My two kids were oblivious to my activity. They had seen it a hundred times before. To their playmates, though, it was all new. They told me they thought parents didn't exercise. "Grown-ups just sit and watch television," they said.

In school, the emphasis is placed on athletics for the gifted few, rather than for everyone. To compound the problem, physical education and athletics generally focus on team sports rather than potential life-long activities such as walking. And what's even worse, participation in school athletics may even discourage future activity. How many times have you seen a coach discipline players by having them run laps or do push-ups as punishment for misbehavior or an error on the athletic field? This punitive approach discourages fitness.

One tragic story involves a young swimmer who won a gold medal in the 1972 Munich Olympics. When he received his last medal, the swimmer vowed never to go back into the pool again. To this day he has refused to do so. When asked to pose with children at a YMCA pool, he said no. He was an Olympic champion, but he missed the boat with respect to lifetime physical activity.

You can help your children build a more positive physical heritage by influencing their activity patterns.

You play an important role when it comes to your children's attitudes about TV and the car. If the TV is on most of the time, your children will learn passive leisure. They will grow up to be armchair quarterbacks. Sometime during the day, assert yourself as a parent and turn off the TV (it's on about five hours, 26 minutes a day in the average American household). While the set is off, encourage walking and other physical activities. Keep the car in the garage. Take it out only when trips really call for it. Less reliance on the car teaches children how to permanently build walking into their lives.

Some families who have tried this have become so wrapped up in walking they now proclaim a "No-Car Day." On that day, no one can use the car except during an emergency.

The Family That Walks Together

Perhaps the best way of all to make walking fun is to make it a family affair. Many people feel that the family is falling apart. Ferdinand Lundberg, author of the *Coming World Transformation,* says, "The family is dead except for the first year or two of child raising." The modern way of life—urbanized, mechanized—is driving each member of the family away from the others. Jobs may force working parents to travel incessantly. The children are in school eight to 10 hours a day. Parents who do not work away from the home may be involved in numerous social functions that keep them busy. As a result, family members don't communicate. There is little touching, little interaction among family members.

Even exercise programs can get in the way of better family relations. Mom and Dad run off to play golf, to a health club, or to tennis lessons. These efforts are nearly useless as ways to attain fitness, and the family suffers because Mom and Dad are again away from the family unit.

Children and parents need an environment that offers touching, talking, sharing, and learning—in other words, better human relations. Dr. Bertram Forer, in the Fall 1969 issue of *Psychotherapy,* notes the need to touch and be touched by other human beings. "The primitive reaction to being touched gently at critical periods is a feeling of body relaxation and assurance that one is not alone, that feelings of unworthiness are not justified." And, he adds, a recent unpublicized poll shows that a majority of clinical psychologists use some forms of physical contact with their patients and have found it significantly useful in treatment. Walking can help overcome these problems. A family walking session can provide a time for touching, talking, sharing, and learning as well as better health.

There is another advantage to walking as a family: motivation. Most of the time, it's difficult for a family to pick an activity that everyone can do well enough so that everyone gets involved. Not everyone has the same skill in tennis, golf or basketball. However, even toddlers can walk, and when they're tired they can be placed in a stroller or baby-sling so Mom and Dad and the older children can keep going.

Next, make sure to vary your route, even if you merely walk in the opposite direction every other day. Or have the children walk the dog or cat (or, perhaps, invite one of their friends). One more thing: let one of the older children lead another child who shuts his or her eyes. (This is an activity that is often used by educators to heighten a child's awareness of his surroundings and his senses.)

Don't push your children into walking. Nagging won't do it. You'll just turn them off. But cooperation, support, and group participation will. Go backpacking or hiking. Walk together to church, to dinner, or to school.

You must emphasize safety. Your children must learn to walk against the traffic. (Every walker has had his own particular harrowing experience when walking with the traffic.) Train your children to walk well off the road and emphasize traffic rules—when to cross at traffic lights, etc. As in driving, they should learn to watch out for the other guy.

Finally, make sure the children wear light-colored clothing. If they are wearing dark clothing, have them wear bright arm bands or hats. That way, motorists can see them better.

We believe you should begin exercising your children as soon as they are born. Dr. Jaroslav Koch, a psychologist, has done extensive work on the relationship between exercise and children's learning patterns. At the Institute of The Care of Mother and Child in Prague, Czechoslovakia, he has shown that children deliberately exercised during the first few months of life have the edge over sedentary children. Their motor development, coordination, and overall physical development are better. And the active child also learns to talk sooner. According to Koch, "The early stimulation of the neuromuscular mechanisms is much more natural than letting the baby lie idly in his cot."

The results of Koch's work are exciting. Get your child exercising; give him the edge in mental, physical, motor, and intellectual development. New moms and dads, buy "papoōse" carriers or slings, put your infant in it, and get moving.

Will you be able to talk your children into walking with you and staying with a walking program? Yes, provided you set an example yourself, and support your children with positive comments. In this way, you'll be able to affect the health and happiness of your family's future generations.

WALKING TOURS

YOU CAN SEE ALL THE SIGHTS AND GET FIT AT THE SAME TIME.

One of the best ways to get to know a city—its people and its flavor—is to get out and walk. Begin with a tour of your own hometown, walk a short portion of your vacation itinerary, take time from business out of town to get to know your host city, or stride out straight from home and walk all the way to your get-away destination.

We've put together a group of tours of some great cities. If we've omitted your favorite, contact a local chamber of commerce for information about city walking sites. Also, a local office of the YMCA in each community may be able to tell you where the city's best walking routes start.

Here is our selection of walking tours. Put one foot in front of the other and enjoy the sights.

Atlanta, Georgia

Downtown. Start at the Atlanta Convention and Visitors Bureau on Peachtree Street, NE. Walk south a few steps to International Boulevard. Turn right and head west toward the Georgia World Congress Center (1), Omni International (2), and the Omni Coliseum. (3). (The Coliseum lies behind Omni International on

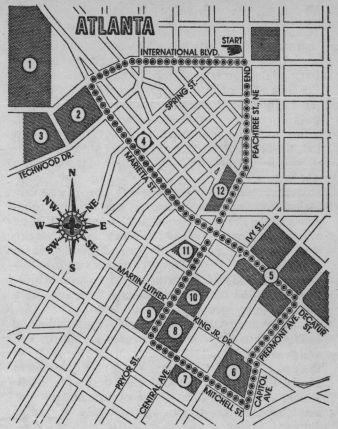

Courtesy of the Atlanta Convention and Visitors Bureau

Atlanta—Map Legend

Start-Atlanta Convention and
Visitors Bureau

(1) Georgia World Congress
    Center

(2) Omni International

(3) Omni Coliseum

(4) Federal Reserve Bank

(5) Georgia State University

(6) Georgia State Capitol

(7) Atlanta City Hall

(8) Fulton County Court House

(9) Shrine of the Immaculate
    Conception

(10) Old Underground Atlanta

(11) Plaza Park

(12) Central City Park

Techwood Drive.) Take a tour if you wish. Then, head southeast on Marietta toward Georgia State University. Along your way, you'll pass the Federal Reserve Bank (4) on your left at Spring Street.

Georgia State University (5) begins at Ivy; the campus will be on both sides of you. At Piedmont Avenue, walk southwest toward the Georgia State Capitol. When you reach Martin Luther King, Jr. Drive, turn left, then right on Capitol Avenue. At Mitchell Street, turn right again. A visit to the Capitol (6) is well worth a stop.

Walking west on Mitchell, you'll see Atlanta City Hall (7) on your left. When you step across Central Avenue, the Fulton County Court House (8) will be on your right. Continue along this block until you get to Pryor Street. Turn right on Pryor and head north. On your left, you'll see the Shrine of the Immaculate Conception (9). Pass over Martin Luther King, Jr. Drive, and you'll find the Atlanta Underground (10) where there are many charming 1890-style stops.

After visiting Old Underground Atlanta, continue heading north on Pryor Street toward Peachtree. You will pass Plaza Park (11) and Central City Park (12). At the end of Central City Park, you'll notice Peachtree Street straight ahead. (Pryor takes a dogleg to the left; Peachtree is to the right.) Once on Peachtree Street, head back to the Atlanta Convention and Visitors Bureau.

For more information, contact the Atlanta Convention and Visitors Bureau, Suite 200, Peachtree Harris Building, 233 Peachtree St., NE, Atlanta, GA 30303; or, Find Your Way In Downtown Atlanta, P.O. Box 8334, Station F, Atlanta, GA 30306.

Baltimore, Maryland

Downtown. Start at the Baltimore Federal Savings and Loan Building (Fayette and St. Paul streets). Walk west on Fayette Street. At Charles Street, turn right.

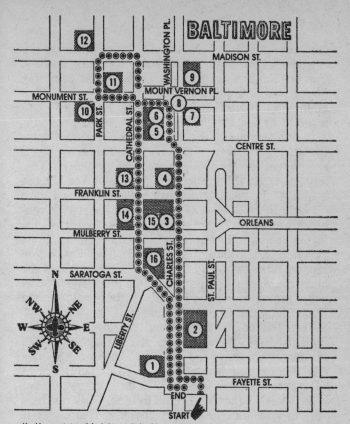

Used by permission of the Baltimore Federal Savings & Loan

Baltimore—Map Legend

Start-Baltimore Federal Savings
and Loan Bldg.

(1) Charles Redevelopment
    Center
(2) St. Paul's Church
(3) Archbishop's Residence
(4) First Unitarian Church
(5) Walters Art Gallery
(6) Gladding House
(7) Peabody Institute
(8) Washington Monument

(9) Mount Vernon Place
    Methodist Church
(10) Maryland Historical Society
(11) St. Peter's Church
(12) First Presbyterian Church
(13) Franklin Street
     Presbyterian Church
(14) Enoch Pratt Free Library
(15) Basilica of the Assumption
(16) St. Paul's Rectory

On your left is the Charles Redevelopment Center (1).
St. Paul's Church (2) is north and to the right of the
Center. Farther north and on the left at Mulberry
Street is the Archbishop's Residence (3). The First
Unitarian Church (1817) (4) is on the corner of Frank-
lin and Charles.

Continue walking north until you get to Centre
Street. Jog left to Washington Place. This is the social
and cultural center of Baltimore. The Walters Art Gallery (5) is on the corner of Centre and Washington
Place. At the end of the block is the Gladding House
(6) built in 1849—one of Baltimore's finest 19th century residences. To your right, at Charles and Washington Street, is the Peabody Institute, the home of the
Peabody Conservatory of Music (7). The Washington
Monument (8) with its 228 steps is in the middle of the
block on Mount Vernon Place. (On the northeast corner of Mount Vernon and Charles is the Mount Vernon
Place Methodist Church (9) built in 1870).

Turn left on Monument and continue walking to
Park. At Park, there are two places to visit. On the
southwest corner is the Maryland Historical Society
(10). There, you will find the original manuscript of
"The Star-Spangled Banner." On the northeast corner
is St. Peter's Church (11) built in 1851. Walk north on
Park to Madison. The First Presbyterian Church (12) is
on the northwest corner. Its 273-foot steeple is the
tallest in Baltimore. Walk east on Madison to Cathedral. Turn right and head south. On the northwest corner of Franklin and Cathedral is the Franklin Street
Presbyterian Church (13). In the next block (right-
hand side) is the Enoch Pratt Free Library (14).
Farther south on the left-hand side is the Basilica of
the Assumption (15). This is the first Roman Catholic
cathedral in the United States.

Continue walking on Cathedral to Saratoga. There,
turn left. On your left, you'll see St. Paul's Rectory
(16) built in 1792. Walk down Saratoga until you come
to Charles Street again. Walk south on Charles to Fay-

ette. Turn left on Fayette to St. Paul. On your right is
the Baltimore Federal Building, your departure point.

For more information, contact the Chamber of Commerce of Metropolitan Baltimore, 22 Light St., Baltimore, MD 21202.

Boston, Massachusetts

Freedom Trail. The Freedom Trail walk begins at the
Freedom Trail Information Center in the Boston Common. Here, you can get free maps and data about the
various historic buildings.

As you follow the red brick line of the Freedom
Trail, you will come to the "new" State House with its
great, gold dome (1). Continue to the Park Street
Church (2) at the corner of Park and Tremont streets.
Next to the church is the Granary Burying Ground (3).
John Hancock, Samuel Adams, Paul Revere, and
other famous revolutionary period people are buried
there.

When you get to School Street, turn right. King's
Chapel (4) is on your left. The chapel was Boston's
first Episcopal church. Now, Unitarian-Universalist
services are held there. The trail will also lead you past
the site of the first public school (Boston Latin School)
(5). On the lawn of the City Hall (6) is a statue of Ben
Franklin.

On the left, where School Street meets Washington
Street, is the Old Corner Bookstore (7)—the famous
literary meeting place of early writers. The old Stone
Meeting House (8) is to your right at the corner of
Washington and Milk streets. (Ben Franklin's birthplace (9) is farther down Milk Street.) Retrace your
steps for half-a-block and continue up Washington
Street to the old State House (10) which was built in
1713. Outside this building is a circle of cobblestones
which marks the site of the Boston Massacre (11).

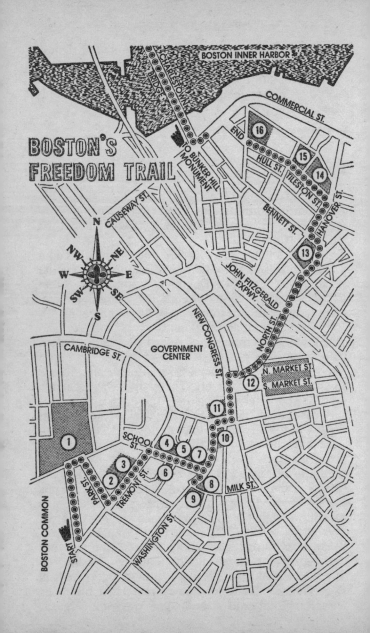

BOSTON'S
FREEDOM TRAIL

BOSTON INNER HARBOR

COMMERCIAL ST.

END

16

15

14

HULL ST.

TILESTON ST.

BENNETT ST.

HANOVER ST.

13

JOHN FITZGERALD EXPWY.

NORTH ST.

CAUSEWAY ST.

TO BUNKER HILL MONUMENT

CHARLESTOWN BRIDGE

N
NW NE
W E
SW SE
S

CAMBRIDGE ST.

GOVERNMENT CENTER

NEW CONGRESS ST.

N. MARKET ST.

S. MARKET ST.

12

11

10

SCHOOL ST.

4

5

7

3

6

2

1

PARK ST

TREMONT ST.

8

9

MILK ST.

BOSTON COMMON

START

WASHINGTON ST.

Boston—Map Legend

Start-Freedom Trail Information
Center

(1) State House	(9) Ben Franklin's Birthplace
(2) Park Street Church	(10) State House
(3) Granary Burying Ground	(11) Boston Massacre Site
(4) King's Chapel	(12) Faneuil Hall
(5) Boston Latin School	(13) Paul Revere's House
(6) City Hall	(14) Paul Revere Mall
(7) Old Corner Bookstore	(15) Old North Church
(8) Stone Meeting House	(16) Copp's Hill Cemetary

Faneuil Hall (12)—the "cradle of liberty"—is your next stop on the Freedom Trail. It faces Quincy Market sandwiched between South and North Market streets. From Faneuil Hall, follow the trail to North Street and the square. There you'll see Paul Revere's house (13). Built in 1666, it's the oldest building in Boston. A short walk from the Revere house by way of Hanover and Tileston streets brings you to the Paul Revere Mall (14) and the Old North Church (15) built in 1723.

You are now in Boston's North End. This is the oldest part of the city, and there is still much to see. Enjoy the sites and the Italian flavor. Up the Hull Street hill to the old church, you'll find Copp's Hill Cemetery (1659) (16). From the burial ground you'll get a good view of Charlestown across the river and the mast of the *U.S.S. Constitution*.

Return to the Common using the red brick route or take the Freedom Trail across the Charlestown Bridge to visit the Bunker Hill Monument and the *Constitution*. (In reality, the monument stands on Breeds Hill, but it commemorates the battle of Bunker Hill.) Monument Avenue takes you to Breeds Hill. Climb the monument's spiral staircase to get a good look at his-

toric Boston. From the Bunker Hill Monument, take
High Street, Adams, Chestnut, Grey, or Water to the
U.S.S. Constitution.

For more information, contact the Division of Tourism, 100 Cambridge St., Boston, MA 02202.

Chicago, Illinois

The Loop. A trip to Chicago wouldn't be complete
without a walking tour of the Loop. Start your tour
facing north at the corner of Monroe and Dearborn.
Walk along Dearborn. To your left will be the First
National Bank Building and Plaza (1) containing the
Chagall mosaic. Continue north to Washington. Turn
left on Washington and head west. On your right,
you'll see the Chicago Civic Center with its Picasso
sculpture (2) and next to it, between Clark and LaSalle
streets, City Hall (3).

Retrace your steps along Washington. On the northeast corner of Washington and State, you'll come to
the Marshall Field and Company Building (4), a noted
Chicago department store. Proceed along Washington
to Wabash and the Elevated, or "El" (5). Pass underneath the El and walk two more blocks past the
Chicago Cultural Center (6).

Turn around and head west on Washington until you
come to State Street again. Turn left and head south.
When you cross Madison, you'll see on your right-hand side the Chicago Building (7) built in 1904 and
Carson Pirie Scott and Company (8) on your left. Continue on to Monroe. There, on the southeast corner,
you'll see the Palmer House (9). Turn right here and
head up Monroe. When you get to Dearborn, turn left
and head south. Soon you'll come to the Marquette
Building (10), an old Chicago landmark. When you do,
turn right and head west on Adams. As you're walking
along Adams, you'll pass the Rookery (11) on the left.

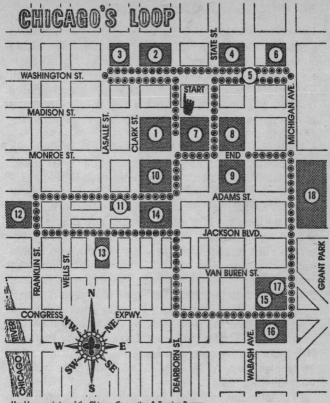

Used by permission of the Chicago Convention & Tourism Bureau

Chicago—Map Legend

Start

(1) First National Bank Bldg. & Plaza
(2) Chicago Civic Center
(3) City Hall
(4) Marshall Field & Co. Bldg.
(5) The Elevated
(6) Chicago Cultural Center
(7) Chicago Bldg.
(8) Carson Pirie Scott & Co.
(9) Palmer House

(10) Marquette Bldg.
(11) Rookery
(12) Sears Tower
(13) Board of Trade Bldg.
(14) Federal Center
(15) Auditorium Bldg.
(16) Pick-Congress Hotel
(17) Fine Arts Bldg.
(18) Art Institute

Continue walking along Adams until you come to Franklin and the world's tallest building, The Sears Tower (12), rising over 1,468 feet into the sky. There is an observation deck 1,350 feet above ground level. This building occupies a full city block and houses over 10,000 employees. It has a power capacity equal to that demanded by Rockford, Illinois, the state's second largest city.

Turn left on Franklin (south) and walk to Jackson. At Jackson, turn left again and head east. Walk under the El at Wells Street; the Board of Trade Building (13) is on your right. You'll also come to the Federal Center (14) which has its entrance on Dearborn. Head south on Dearborn for a few blocks. You'll pass under the El again at Van Buren. Continue down to Congress. Turn left on Congress. As you do, you'll pass the Auditorium Building (15) and the Pick-Congress Hotel (16) on your left and right, respectively. Each of these have their entrances on South Michigan Avenue.

At Michigan Avenue turn left and head north. To your left is the Fine Arts Building (17) built in 1884. On your right is Grant Park containing The Art Institute (18) (between Jackson and Monroe). It's worth a walk on another day. At Monroe turn left and head back to your starting point.

(You also have another alternative. At Monroe you can take a right and head out to the Monroe Street Harbor and Chicago's Lakefront.)

For further information, contact the Chicago Convention and Tourism Bureau, 332 S. Michigan Ave., Suite 2000, Chicago, IL 60611 or Chicago Center Area Committee, 111 West Washington Ave., Chicago, IL 60602.

Cleveland, Ohio

Emerald Necklace. The Cleveland Metroparks are a series of 11 parks bordering three sides of the city with

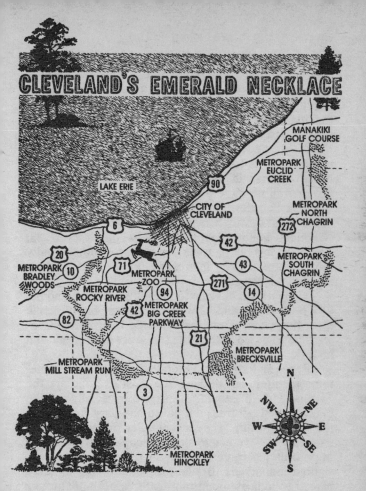

CLEVELAND'S EMERALD NECKLACE

MANAKIKI GOLF COURSE

METROPARK EUCLID CREEK

LAKE ERIE

CITY OF CLEVELAND

METROPARK NORTH CHAGRIN

METROPARK SOUTH CHAGRIN

METROPARK BRADLEY WOODS

METROPARK ROCKY RIVER

METROPARK ZOO

METROPARK BIG CREEK PARKWAY

METROPARK MILL STREAM RUN

METROPARK BRECKSVILLE

METROPARK HINCKLEY

N
NW NE
W   E
SW SE
S

a lush, green landscape. It is for this reason that the
system is called the "Emerald Necklace." There are
18,000 acres of parks situated about 15 miles from
downtown. Some are located in the city itself, but
most are to be found in the neighboring suburbs.

Metropark Rocky River is located to the west of the
city. This huge 5,680 acre park has many entrances.
Detroit Avenue in the Lakewood area, Rockcliff Road

in the Rocky River area, and Eastland Road in Middlesburgh Heights are only three. For the walker, there's a Trailside Interpretive Center, a waterfowl sanctuary, fascinating geological exposures, picnic facilities, and bike trails. (A 5-mile paved trail goes from Detroit Avenue (Lakewood) to Old Lorain Road.) At the Rocky River Trailside Interpretive Center, naturalists take walkers along five miles of trails. Most walkers will also delight in the well marked wildflower trail near the South Mastick picnic area. West 220 near Fairview Park will get you there.

Metropark Mill Stream Run to the southwest of Cleveland can be entered from West 30th St. or Rt. 82. This park has hiking trails that take you along rapidly moving streams, by interesting flood plains, and up and down steep slopes.

Metropark Brecksville to the south of Cleveland between routes 21 and 82 warrants a visit. Many scenic trails branch out from the Trailside Interpretive Center. The trails along the Ohio Canal are both scenic and historic.

All these parks in the Emerald Necklace have something to offer, but perhaps the most exciting are the "Trails For All People." Designed especially for the handicapped, all trails are paved and vary from six to ten feet in width. They are circular or follow a loop pattern and have gentle slopes. People in wheelchairs or on crutches can easily use the trails. To assist nonsighted individuals, Braille plaques are appropriately placed to indicate important features of the nature or history in a particular area. Also, the Interpretive Center at Rocky River offers a unique trail guide for the deaf. These truly are "Trails For All People."

For more information, contact the Greater Cleveland Growth Association, 690 Union St., Commerce Building, Cleveland, OH 44115; or Cleveland Metroparks, 55 Public Square, Cleveland, OH 44113.

Dallas, Texas

Big D Tours. Big D has a b-i-g park system—more than 14,000 acres. Near downtown is the Cotton Bowl and State Fair Park, to the southeast off I-45 is Rochester Park, and to the northeast off I-35E you'll find Elm Fork Park. In the northeast corner is White Rock Lake Park surrounding White Rock Lake.

Try the nature trails on the west side of the city. Take your choice of five walks that range in duration from a half hour to more than two hours, depending upon the course you take. The most interesting of the walks is the lower section of the Wilderness Way along the Trinity River.

For more information, contact Dallas Convention and Visitors Bureau, Dallas Chamber of Commerce, 1507 Pacific Ave., Dallas, TX 75201.

Denver, Colorado

Downtown Denver. Start your tour at 225 West Colfax Avenue—the Convention and Visitors Bureau of Denver and Colorado. It has complete visitor information, including maps and brochures. Walk east on East Colfax Avenue to the State Capitol Complex (1). The complex is bounded by Broadway on the west, Grant Street on the east, East Colfax Avenue to the north, and East 13th Avenue to the south. Included here are the State Capitol Building, State Services Building, State Office Building, and State Annex. The Colorado Capitol Building is a must. It is constructed of grey granite patterned after the United States Capitol in Washington, D.C. The 13th step on the west side is marked by a plaque. It is exactly one mile above sea level. The capitol's gold dome is a memorial to Colorado's mining industry. Be sure to visit the dome

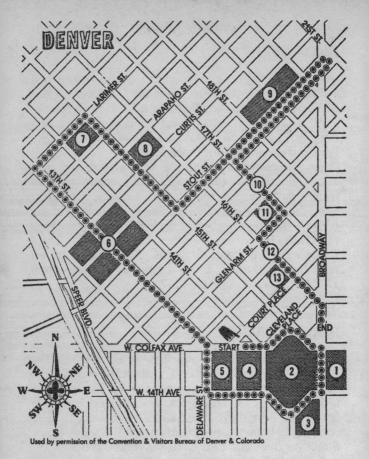

Denver—Map Legend

Start-
Convention and Visitors Bureau
of Denver & Colorado

(1) State Capitol Complex

(2) Civic Center

(3) Denver Public Library

(4) City and County Bldg.

(5) United States Mint

(6) Denver Convention
    Complex and Center for
    the Performing Arts

(7) Larimer Square

(8) Federal Reserve Bank

(9) Federal Complex

(10) Wall Street of the West

(11) Eisenhower Chapel

(12) 16th St. Shopping Center

(13) Court Place Plaza

gallery. The view from it is magnificent. To the west lie the Rockies and to the east, the Great Plains.

Leave the capitol by the west exit and stride toward the Civic Center (2). The Center is a three-block area that includes beautifully manicured lawns and gardens. The Denver Public Library is here, along with an outdoor Greek theater, fountains, and monuments to Colorado pioneers (3). Next to the library, at East 13th Street and Broadway, is the Colorado Heritage Center, the headquarters of the Colorado Historical Society.

After your visit, strike out west on 14th Avenue. On your right will be the City and County Building (4). When you get to Delaware, turn right. The entrance to the United States Mint is on Delaware Avenue (5).

When you reach West Colfax Avenue, walk northwest up 13th Street. At Stout Street, you'll come to the Denver Convention Complex and Center for the Performing Arts (6). Here, you'll find the 100,000-square-foot Currigan Exhibition Hall and various theater buildings. Continue on 13th, turn right on Larimer Street, and continue to Larimer Square (7), a private renewal area within Denver's downtown urban renewal project. (Larimer was a famous street in the frontier West.) Shops, restaurants, night spots, and galleries with a mid-Victorian flavor dot this area. The gaslights and courtyards reflect the same period.

At 15th Street, turn right and proceed southwest. Between Arapaho and Curtis, you'll come to the Federal Reserve Bank (8). Continue down 15th Street, turn left on Stout Street, and walk to the area between 18th and 21st streets. There, you'll find a Federal complex (9) including a United States Post Office, the United States Court Building, a new Customs House, and the Federal Power Building.

Retrace your steps to 17th Street and turn left. Proceed on 17th Street to the area between Arapaho and Broadway. This is considered the Wall Street of the West (10). Many major banks, investment and brokerage houses are here. The Eisenhower Chapel is on

17th and Glenarm Place (11). Turn right on Glenarm and walk to the 16th Street shopping center (between Cleveland Place and Arapaho) (12). The district is Denver's primary downtown shopping area. It includes many department stores, specialty shops, theaters, and restaurants.

Now that you're on 16th Street, proceed southwest to the Court Place Plaza (13). Here, you'll find ice skating in the winter and a sculptured garden in the summer. Continue along 16th Street till you come to Broadway. Turn right and walk along Broadway to Colfax Avenue. You can turn right here and go back to your starting point, or if you're ambitious you might head east on Colfax until you come to Pennsylvania Street. Turn right on Pennsylvania and walk toward the district of Victorian homes. At 1340 Pennsylvania Street, there is an unusual house which was once the home of the "unsinkable" heiress, Molly Brown. Other ornate Victorian homes can be seen on your way to 9th Avenue. Turn around at 9th Avenue and return to East Colfax Avenue, your point of departure.

For more information, contact the Denver Chamber of Commerce, 1301 Welton St., Denver, CO 80204; or Convention and Visitors Bureau, 225 W. Colfax, Denver, CO 80202.

Detroit, Michigan

Detroit tours. Detroit's park system covers about 6,000 acres and includes more than 200 parks and playgrounds. Belle Isle is a 982-acre park right in the middle of the Detroit River, only four miles from downtown. It has good walking courses, an aquarium, a beach, and a children's zoo. Chandler Park is at the Edsel Ford Freeway and Connor. Palmer Park is only four miles from downtown and near the University of Detroit. It is also near the State Fairgrounds. Rouge

Park, the largest of all in the Detroit area, comprises 1,172 acres. It includes a golf course, swimming pool, tennis courts, and many pleasant paths.

For more information, contact Detroit Chamber of Commerce, 150 Michigan Ave., Detroit, MI 48226.

Honolulu, Hawaii

Island City Walks. Start your Honolulu walking tour at the Kamehameha statue on Mililani Street. Proceed west to Merchant Street, which takes you past the post office facing Richards Street. Go north on Richards Street to King Street. There, turn left and head east. The YMCA will be on your right. At Fort Street, walk south toward the ocean, passing Merchant Street and Nimitz Highway. As Fort Street turns left, it becomes Ala Moana Boulevard. On the right, see the Aloha Tower at Pier 9 and the waterfront. The Tower provides a good view of the harbor and the city.

Leaving Pier 9, head for Pier 5 and board the *Falls of Clyde*. This 100-year-old, four-masted, fully rigged ship is being restored by the Bishop Museum. After a visit to the ship, walk north toward the buildings of the State Civic Center Mall. Here, you'll find the Federal Building and the United States Courthouse. These unique, low-slung structures are well worth a visit. Next, head left toward Bishop Street. Take it north to Hotel Street.

Turn left on Hotel and stride east into Chinatown. At Maunakea Street, you'll see the pagoda-like restaurant called Wo Fat. Continue walking west on Hotel to River Street. Stroll up and down River Street: The fish market is down near Nimitz Highway; the wholesale produce market and Lumsai Ho Tong (Taoist temple) are at the north end of River. Enjoy Chinatown and its shops. At west River Street and Beretania, you'll see the Japanese hotel, Kobayashi, facing Aala Park.

After you have visited this blend of oriental cultures, go back to Hotel Street, swing left, and proceed east. On your way, you'll pass the Armed Forces YMCA on your left. Iolani Palace, until recently the state capitol, is on your right. It is the only royal palace on American soil. The archives are to the east of the palace. On the corner of Hotel and Punchbowl streets, you'll find the library. Take Punchbowl Street south. At King Street, you'll see the City Hall on your left. Turn left on King to Alapai Street, then left again. This will take you past the new Honolulu Municipal Building. When you get to Beretania Street, turn left. You'll pass the Board of Water Supply and the State Office Building. When you reach Punchbowl Street again, go south toward King Street. On the southeast corner are the Kawaia Hao Church Mission Houses, once visited by Hawaiian royalty. From the church, retrace your steps along King Street to the Kamehameha statue.

For more information, contact the Chamber of Commerce of Hawaii, 735 Bishop St., Honolulu, HI 96813.

Houston, Texas

Texas Trek. Houston has many different and fascinating places to visit including 200 parks and playgrounds that cover about 5,000 acres. Hermann Park, about three miles south of downtown (on Main Street), includes the Houstonian Zoological Gardens. You'll also find the children's zoo and the Municipal Rose Garden there. In the same area are the Museum of Natural Science, the Museum of Fine Arts, and the Contemporary Arts Museum.

In Sam Houston Park you'll see what the city looked like in the 1800s. Memorial Park, to the west of the city and bounded by I-10 on the north and I-610 to the west, has nature trails, picnic areas, swimming pools, and horse paths.

Of course, you don't have to confine your efforts to the park areas. There are places to walk downtown, too. The Houston Chamber of Commerce suggests that you get two walking guides for the Houston area. They are *Step-By-Step* and *Intrepid Walker's Guide To Houston;* both are available at your book store.

For more information, contact the Houston Chamber of Commerce, 25th Floor, 1100 Meilam Building, Houston, TX 77002.

Los Angeles, California

Walking L.A. Los Angeles has more than 200 parks and similar recreational facilities. Griffith Park is the largest city-owned and city-operated park in the world with its more than 4,000 acres and 50 miles of horse trails. The park also contains the Los Angeles Zoo and the Griffith Observatory and Planetarium.

Santa Monica Beach and the sidewalks over Redondo Beach are other good places to walk. Still others include Hollywood Park (near the airport); Exposition Park, which contains the Museum of Natural History, the Memorial Coliseum, and the Museum of Science and Industry; and the University of Southern California. Elysia Park is near Dodger Stadium.

For more information, contact the Los Angeles Area Chamber of Commerce, 404 South Bixel St., Los Angeles, CA 90017.

Miami, Florida

Parks. Except at the height of the hot, humid summer, Miami is a perfect place to walk. Greynolds Park at the north end (northeast 179th Street and northeast 22nd

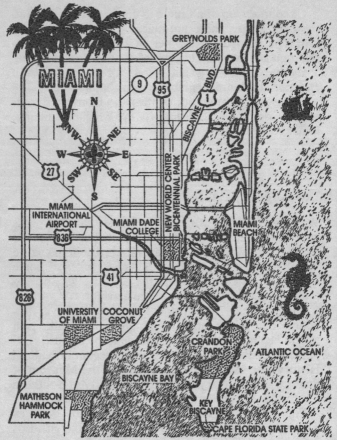

Avenue) is especially good on Sundays when cars are forbidden access.

Crandon Park in Key Biscayne is excellent. So, too, are Cape Florida State Park and Matheson Hammock Park near Coral Gables. The treelined streets of Coral Gables, the campuses of the University of Miami and Miami Dade Community College South and New

World Center Bicentennial Park are additional good places to walk.

For more information, contact the Greater Miami Chamber of Commerce, Biscayne Blvd., Miami, FL 33132. Ask for information regarding free monthly walking tours through the coconut groves. The tours start at Peacock Park across from the Coconut Grove Library at 2875 McFarlane Road.

Milwaukee, Wisconsin

Downtown. Start your tour at the Greater Milwaukee Convention and Visitors Bureau, Inc. Proceed north on Broadway to Kilbourn Avenue. Turn left. Walk along Kilbourn; at Water Street, turn right. On the left-hand side, at 929 North Water Street, is the Performing Arts Center (1).

Visit the center, then move north to State Street. Turn left on State and cross over the Milwaukee River. Between 4th and 6th avenues, you'll come to the MECCA Complex, an auditorium, arena and convention hall (2). Farther on and to your right, you will find the Milwaukee Area Technical College (3). Continue walking along State to 9th Street. There, turn right to Highland. Directly in front of you is the Pabst Brewing Company (4). Circle the block to the main entrance at 901 West Juneau Avenue.

After a refreshing tour, walk right along Juneau Avenue back to 7th Street. Turn right and go south. At West Kilbourn Avenue, you'll come to the Civic Center Plaza (5). Included among the public buildings to the right and left are the County Courthouse, the Public Safety Building, a museum and state office buildings and MECCA. Turn left along West Kilbourn Avenue to Broadway; turn south and return to your original point of departure.

For further information, contact the Greater Milwaukee Convention and Visitors Bureau, Inc., 828 N. Broadway, Milwaukee, WI 53202.

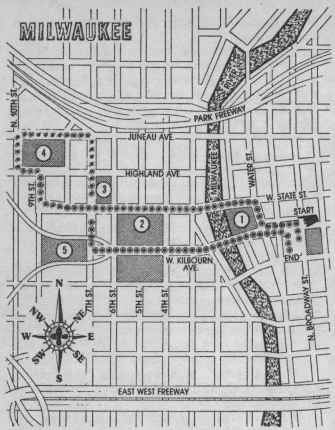

Used by permission of the Greater Milwaukee Convention & Visitors Bureau

Milwaukee—Map Legend

Start-Greater Milwaukee
Convention and Visitors
Bureau, Inc.

(1) Performing Arts Center

(2) MECCA Complex

(3) Milwaukee Area Technical
College

(4) Pabst Brewing Co.

(5) Civic Center Plaza

Minneapolis/St. Paul, Minnesota

Twin Cities Tours. There are many places to walk in the Twin Cities. Minneapolis has almost 150 parks that encompass 5,500 acres. Most of them line the Mississippi River or the lakes in the city. The largest is Theodore Worth Park at the west end. Its 740 acres are perfect for slow walking or hiking. Lake Nokomis Park has a three and a half mile trail encircling it. You can get there by traveling west on Olsen Memorial Highway or by taking US-12, also known as the Wayzata Boulevard. Just to the south of Theodore Worth Park is Lake Calhoun and Lake Harriet. A walk around both of these lakes is almost seven miles. North of Lake Nokomis Park is Hiawatha Park with a lake of the same name. This park sprawls eastward and becomes Minnehaha Park. It contains the 53-foot Minnehaha Falls. All three parks are perfect places for a walk.

Across the Mississippi are still more walking areas. Lake Como in Como Park at Hamline and Como avenues contains the city zoo. Phelan Park surrounds Lake Phelan. You can get to it by taking Larpenteur Avenue or Maplewood Drive. To the south of Phelan Park are Indian Mounds Park and Battle Creek Park.

For more information, contact Minnesota Vacations, 51 East 8th St., St. Paul, MN 55101.

Montreal, Quebec
Canada

Montreal Tours. There's good walking in Montreal. One place to go is Old Montreal which borders the St. Lawrence River between Berri and McGill streets. Here, old buildings nestle next to tall, modern structures. Restaurants, historic houses, and small retail shops line Old Montreal's narrow streets, some of which are paved with cobblestones. In this area, the city's oldest church, Notre Dame de Bon Secours, stands on St. Paul Street. The church was built in 1771 on the foundation of an older building. Some people call it The Sailors' Church. It forms the northern boundary of Old Montreal.

At the southern end of this area on Notre Dame Street is St. Sulpice Seminary, housed in the oldest building in Montreal. It was opened in 1685. Near the seminary are two historic squares. Across Notre Dame Street is the Parade Ground, where the first clash between the city's founders and the Iroquois Indians took place in 1644. East of the seminary on St. Paul Street is Royal Square. This square is the site of Fort Montreal built in 1642.

For further information, contact City of Montreal, 2, Place Ville-Marie, Montreal, Quebec, Canada.

Nashville, Tennessee

Nashville Tours. Start at Fort Nashborough overlooking the Cumberland River. Stop for a visit, then go north (right) on First Avenue. At Church Street, turn left. At Second Avenue is the Second Avenue Historic District consisting of a group of Victorian commercial buildings (1). At Union Street, turn left. On your left you'll see the Stahlman Building (2) and the American Trust Building (3) built in 1926. Farther on the right are the First American Bank (4) and the new Commerce Place (5).

At Fourth Avenue, walk south. On the right, you will see the Arcade (6)—one of the first covered shopping areas in the United States. At the corner of Church and Fourth are four interesting buildings: the United American Bank (7), Nashville's first skyscraper (12 stories), on the northeast corner; the J. C. Bradford Building (8) on the southeast corner; the Life and Casualty Tower (with observation deck) (9) on the

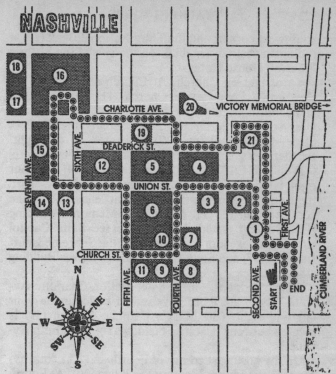

Used by permission of the Historical Commission of Metropolitan Nashville and Davidson County

Nashville—Map Legend

Start-Fort Nashborough

(1) Second Avenue Historic
District
(2) Stahlman Bldg.
(3) American Trust Bldg.
(4) First American Bank
(5) Commerce Place
(6) Arcade
(7) United American Bank
(8) J.C. Bradford Bldg.
(9) Life and Casualty Tower
(10) Third National Bank
(11) Downtown Presbyterian
Church

(12) Performing Arts Center
(13) Hermitage Hotel
(14) Hyatt-Regency Hotel
(15) War Memorial Bldg.
(16) Tennessee State Capitol
(17) Supreme Court Bldg.
(18) State Library and Archives
Bldg.
(19) St. Mary's Catholic Church
(20) Morris Memorial Bldg.
(21) Metropolitan
Nashville-Davidson County
Courthouse

southwest corner; and the Third National Bank (10) at the northwest corner, built on the site of the historic Maxwell House Hotel.

Turn right on Church. At Church and Fifth is the Downtown Presbyterian Church (11) built in 1851. Head north (right) up Fifth, then left at Union. At Union the new Performing Arts Center (James K. Polk Street Office Building) (12) is located on the right. Farther west on the left side are the Hermitage Hotel (13) built in 1910 and the Hyatt-Regency (14). On your right is the Tennessee Government Complex. Turn right and walk along the plaza that leads you to the complex. On the left is the War Memorial Building (15). Straight ahead is the Tennessee State Capitol (16). To the west of the capitol are the Supreme Court Building (17) and State Library and Archives Building (18).

After visiting this area, walk east on Charlotte Avenue. There are more government buildings on your left and right. (St. Mary's Catholic Church (19) is located between tall office buildings south on Fifth Avenue.)

On the northeast corner of Fourth and Charlotte avenues is the Morris Memorial Building (20). At Fourth Avenue, turn right and then left at Deaderick Street. Straight ahead is the old Public Square. In the center of the square is the Metropolitan Nashville-Davidson County Courthouse (21). From here go south on Second Avenue; take Church Street to First Avenue to get back to your starting point.

For more information, contact the Nashville Chamber of Commerce, 161 Fourth Ave. North, Nashville, TN 37219.

New Orleans, Louisiana

French Quarter. Start at the Decatur Moon Walk. While there, take in the beautiful view of the Mississippi River. The Greater New Orleans Bridge (1958) is on your right. Jackson Square is behind you, and, farther on, the St. Louis Cathedral. Leaving the Moon Walk area, turn right on Decatur and walk east. Veer right onto French Market Street (1). At Barracks is the old United States Mint (2), the site of Fort St. Charles in 1815. Walk left on Barracks to Chartres. Turn left. On your right is The Barracks (3) built in 1757. At Governor Nicholls turn right and walk up to Royal Street. On the corner of Governor Nicholls and Royal is The Haunted House (4). A woman by the name of Delphine LaLaurie starved and tortured her slaves there. The house burned in 1835. It was rebuilt, but people say that the slaves still haunt it.

Turn left and walk along Royal. At 915 is The Royal Cornstalk Fence (5). At 908, you'll see the back of the beautiful Miltenberger mansions, built by a widow for her three sons (6). At Dumaine, turn left and walk south. At 632 is one of the oldest buildings in the Mississippi Valley (1726), now a state museum (7). Retrace your steps to Royal; turn left. At St. Ann and Royal is the Languille Building (8), the tallest building in New Orleans when it was built in 1801.

At Orleans, turn right and walk north. You'll see the Orleans Ballroom (9) at 717. Some of the most fashionable dances of the 1800s were held there. Turn left at Bourbon Street then left on St. Peter. (Preservation Hall (10) is on this street.) At Royal Street, turn right. Patty's Court (11), an attractive courtyard, is at 631; the home of Zachary Taylor, 12th U.S. president (12), is at 621 Royal; and the French Governor's Home (13) is at 615 Royal. Farther on down the street, you'll come to the Court of Two Lions (14), another home with a beautiful courtyard.

When you reach St. Louis Street, turn right. Antoine's (15), the oldest restaurant in New Orleans, is on St. Louis. At Bourbon Street, walk to your right. The street widens at 541, the site of the Old French Opera House (16). Here, the carriages stopped to let their passengers disembark.

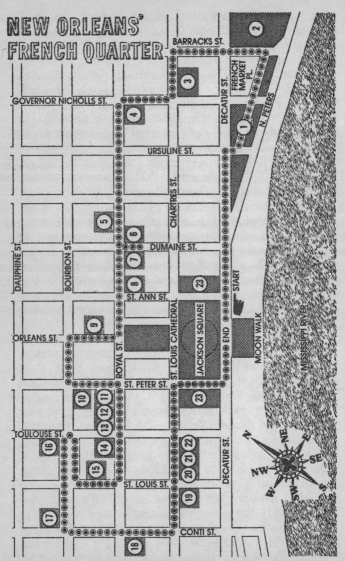

Used by permission of the Greater New Orleans Tourist & Convention Commission

New Orleans—Map Legend

Start-Decatur Moon Walk

(1) French Market Street
(2) Old United States Mint
(3) The Barracks
(4) The Haunted House
(5) Royal Cornstalk Fence
(6) Miltenberger Mansion
(7) State Museum
(8) Languille Bldg.
(9) Orleans Ballroom
(10) Preservation Hall
(11) Patty's Court
(12) Zachary Taylor's Home
(13) French Governor's Home

(14) Court of Two Lions
(15) Antoine's
(16) Old French Opera House
(17) Old Absinthe Bar
(18) Greater New Orleans
     Tourist & Convention
     Commission
(19) Maspero's Exchange
(20) Napoleon House
(21) Pharmaceutical Museum
(22) 1788 Fire
(23) Pontabla Bldg.

Turn around and walk back along Bourbon. On the northeast corner of Bourbon and Conti is the old Absinthe Bar (17). Turn left on Conti. The intersection of Conti and Royal—with a bank on each corner—was the financial hub of New Orleans years ago. The Old Bank of Louisiana (at 334 Royal) is now the Greater New Orleans Tourist Convention Commission (18).

Proceed south on Conti to Chartres Street. Turn left and walk back toward Jackson Square. At 440 Chartres is Maspero's Exchange (19), an early coffee house. Farther up the street (at 500) is the Napoleon House (20), a home offered to but unoccupied by the exiled emperor. Farther along is the Pharmaceutical Museum (21) with displays of medical and voodoo implements of the 1800s. At 538 Chartres is the site of the start of the 1788 fire (22) which destroyed 856 buildings in New Orleans. Turn right at St. Peter and walk past Jackson Square. To your right is the Pontabla Building (23). A sister building is on the opposite side of Jackson Square.

Jackson Square was originally designed as a drill field. In the 1800s it was converted into a park. A statue of Andrew Jackson now graces the grounds.

For further information, contact New Orleans Chamber of Commerce, P.O. Box 30240, New Orleans, LA 70190.

New York, New York

Greenwich Village. The Village is bounded by 14th Street on the north, Houston Street on the south, Hudson Street on the west (although some say it extends to the river), and Lafayette Street on the east. The center of the Village is Washington Square. At the western end—Washington Square West—is MacDougal Street. Walk up MacDougal Street to MacDougal Alley (1). At one time, these tiny homes were stables and carriage houses. Numbers 27 and 131 MacDougal were built for Aaron Burr in the early 1800s. Some of the oldest buildings in the city are here.

Retrace your steps on MacDougal. You'll come to Minetta Lane (2), a street named after Minetta Brook, which now runs underground.

MacDougal Street crosses Bleeker. Detour down the block, between Bleeker and Houston, to see some neat, old brick homes, then walk back to Bleeker and turn left. Head up on Bleeker Street toward LeRoy Street. Turn left on LeRoy toward St. Luke's Place. (Both of these roads wind quite a bit.) At St. Luke's, you'll see some attractive Italian-style houses along a treelined street (3). These were built in the 1800s.

Turn right on Hudson and take your pick of the various twisting, turning streets to explore Greenwich Village. Morton Street is fun. Turn right and enjoy it up to Bedford. Turn left.

At 75½ Bedford, you'll find the narrowest house in all of New York. Only 9 feet wide, it was built in the driveway of an old farmhouse. Next door, at 77 Bedford Street, is the oldest house in the city. At the corner of Bedford and Grove are other interesting houses (4)—a historic mansion with almost doll-house-size

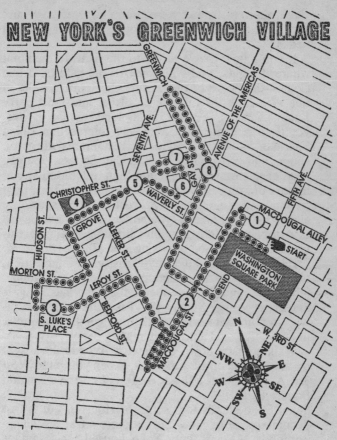

Used by permission of Nester's Map & Guide Corp.

New York—Map Legend

Start-Washington Square West

(1) MacDougal Alley

(2) Minetta Lane

(3) Italian-Style Houses

(4) Interesting Houses

(5) Sheridan Square

(6) Greek-Style Houses

(7) Browsing Area

(8) Village Square

slave quarters from several hundred years ago and another house, at 100 Bedford, known as "Twin Peaks."

If you follow Grove Street to the right, to the point where it bends, you will come to the gate of Grove Court—the home of the writer, O. Henry. (While in this area look for Commerce Street and the Cherry Lane Theater.) As you walk northeast on Grove, you'll soon come to a nine-way intersection called Sheridan Square (5). Here are restaurants, theaters, shops, and cafes. Once at Sheridan Square, you can head back toward Washington Square Park on Washington, or you can walk to Waverly Place. Turn right on Waverly and left on Gay Street, an interesting little alley with many Greek-type homes (6). Follow Gay to Christopher Street. Once on Christopher, angle westward. Here is a good browsing area (7).

Backtracking past the Gay-Christopher intersection, turn right to the intersection of Greenwich Avenue, 8th Street, and the Avenue of the Americas. This is known as Village Square (8). Take Greenwich northwest for an interesting walk past good restaurants, unique cafes, and among interesting people.

Walking back down Greenwich Avenue, turn right on the Avenue of the Americas. When you get to West 3rd Avenue, turn left and walk back to Washington Square Park.

Soho. Soho stands for "south of Houston." It is fast becoming one of New York's most attractive neighborhoods. At one time, Soho housed the infamous "sweat shops" of the city. Today, it serves New York's art community. There are dozens of good galleries, new restaurants, and shops to enjoy. On weekends, Soho is an outdoor cultural center as artists display their wares along the walks.

For further information, contact Downtown-Lower Manhattan Association, Inc., 61 Broadway, New York, NY 10006.

Philadelphia, Pennsylvania

A History Tour. Start at City Hall at the center of Broad Street. Proceed east on Market Street toward Independence Park. As you walk along Market Street, you will pass the Reading Terminal at 12th Street (1). Farther on, between 8th and 10th streets, you'll come to the Gallery Mall (2). Both of these are on your left.

At 6th Street, you'll come to the United States Courthouse (3). Turn right on 6th and walk to Chestnut. To your left will be Independence National Park (4), bordered by Chestnut and Walnut, 5th and 6th. In this area, you'll get a real lesson in American history. Congress Hall (5) is at 6th and Chestnut streets. Between 5th and 6th streets on Chestnut is Independence Hall (6). Behind Independence Hall, you'll see the Liberty Bell Pavilion (7). Old City Hall (8) is located at 5th and Chestnut streets. Liberty Hall (9) is at 5th Street just below Chestnut Street, and the Second Bank of the United States (10) is on Chestnut Street between 4th and 5th streets.

To the east of the Second Bank between 3rd and 4th streets on Chestnut is the Army-Navy Museum (11). The Marine Corps Museum is in the same area (12), and Carpenter Hall (13) is at 3rd and Chestnut streets. Immediately behind Carpenter Hall is the First Bank of the United States (14), and behind that is the Philadelphia Merchant Exchange (15).

If you feel like extending your walk, you can go back up 3rd Street to Market. Swing right on Market and head toward the Delaware River. At the end of Market Street and under I-95 you'll come to Penn's Landing at Delaware Avenue (16). This runs from Race to Lombard Street. At the southern end of Penn's Landing, you will find the *U.S.S. Olympia* (17). Retrace your steps to Market Street, then turn left and walk to Front Street. Take it (right) to Elfreth's Alley (18), only a few blocks north. This is a house-lined,

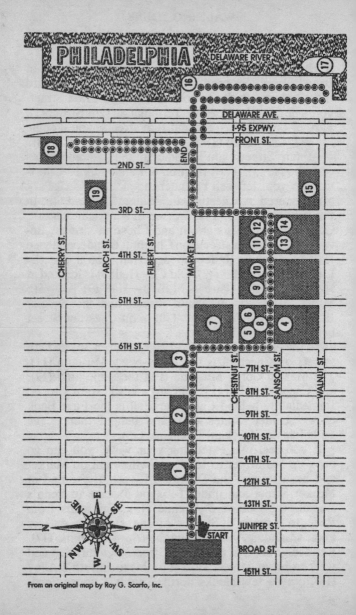

Philadelphia—Map Legend

Start-City Hall

(1) Reading Terminal
(2) Gallery Mall
(3) United States Courthouse
(4) Independence National Park
(5) Congress Hall
(6) Independence Hall
(7) Liberty Bell Pavilion
(8) Old City Hall
(9) Liberty Hall
(10) Second Bank of the U.S.

(11) Army-Navy Museum
(12) Marine Corps Museum
(13) Carpenter Hall
(14) First Bank of the United States
(15) Philadelphia Merchant Exchange
(16) Penn's Landing
(17) U.S.S. Olympia
(18) Elfreth's Alley
(19) Betsy Ross House

---

cobblestone lane dating back to 1702. The Betsy Ross house (19) is near this area. To get back to your starting point, simply retrace your steps or catch public transportation.

For further information, contact Philadelphia Chamber of Commerce, 1528 Walnut St., Philadelphia, PA 19102.

Pittsburgh, Pennsylvania

Golden Triangle. Start at Point State Park and proceed into the city toward the Crosstown Boulevard. Walking in this direction, you pass such famous buildings as Mellon's National Bank, the United States Steel Building, Alcoa Building, Mellon Square Park, Trinity Church, Pines Hall, and the Equitable Plaza.

There are 36 parks in Pittsburgh with paths. One walk is in the north hills around North Park Lake, which covers more than five miles. In Schenley Park there is a 10,000-meter bike trail.

Another good place to walk is Pittsburgh's Oakland area, including three colleges: The University of Pittsburgh, Carlow College, and Carnegie-Mellon University.

For further information, contact Pittsburgh Chamber of Commerce, Chamber of Commerce Bldg., Pittsburgh, PA 15219.

Portland, Oregon

Portland Tours. Start at the Portland Center on SW Market Street. This attractive complex of apartments and offices with wide walkways, plazas, shops, trees, and the Lovejoy Fountain is a great beginning. Take SW 2nd Street to SW Clay and turn left. The Civic Auditorium (1) is at 222 SW Clay. In the next block, between SW 3rd and SW 4th, you'll find Ira's Fountain (2). Thirteen thousand gallons of water a minute pour over a waterfall 18 feet high and 80 feet wide.

Proceed north on SW Clay to SW Ninth. On your left is Portland State University (3). Turn right and walk toward the Portland Arts Museum (4), the Sculpture Mall (5) at SW Madison, the Museum Art School (6), and Farrell's Sycamore (7) located at Main Street. This giant sycamore, now a Portland landmark, was planted nearly 100 years ago. Walk to SW Taylor. Turn left and head north. Turn right on SW 10th. Soon, you'll come to a Benson's Drinking Fountain (8), one of several built during Prohibition. Continue walking on SW 10th to SW Morrison. Turn right onto Morrison and left onto 9th. On your left, at SW 9th and Adler, is the Galleria (9), a shopping mall with 46 shops and restaurants on many levels. It's an exciting and interesting place to visit. Continue walking along SW 9th to O'Bryant Square at SW Washington (10). The unusual open-brick plaza is a fascinating place to walk around.

From the square, walk right on SW Washington toward the Willamette River. On your right is Morgan's Alley (11), an arcade that cuts through the Morgan Building from Broadway to Park and from Washington

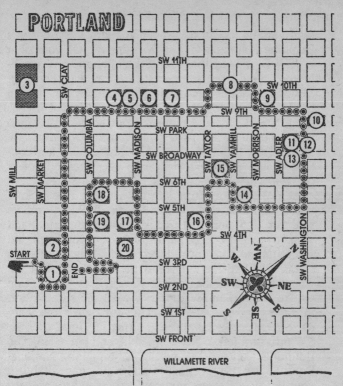

Used by permission of the Greater Portland Convention and Visitors Association

Portland—Map Legend

Start-Portland Center

(1) Civic Auditorium
(2) Ira's Fountain
(3) Portland State University
(4) Portland Arts Museum
(5) Sculpture Mall
(6) Museum Art School
(7) Farrell's Sycamore
(8) Benson's Drinking Fountain
(9) Galleria
(10) O'Bryant Square
(11) Morgan's Alley

(12) Benson's Drinking Fountain
(13) Cast-Iron Street Clocks
(14) Pioneer Courthouse
(15) Jackson Tower
(16) Georgia-Pacific Bldg.
(17) Standard Plaza (Ring of Time)
(18) Equitable Center
(19) First National Bank Tower
(20) Schrunk Plaza

to Adler streets. Stop for a sip at another of Benson's
Drinking Fountains (12) on Washington. On your right
on SW Broadway (between SW Adler and SW Washington), you'll see some cast-iron street clocks (13).
Continue walking toward the river on SW Washington
until you come to SW 5th. There, turn right. On your
right, you'll pass the Pioneer Courthouse (14) which
was built in 1873. Turn right at the corner of SW
Yamhill and proceed toward SW 6th; turn left and continue walking. On your right will be the Jackson Tower
(15) with its four-sided clock.

At SW Taylor, turn left toward the river. Soon
you'll come to the Georgia-Pacific Building and its
sculpture (16) built in 1970. At SW 4th, turn right and
stop to visit the Logging Museum and underground
sculpture on the lower level of the Georgia-Pacific
Building. Take the tunnel to the historical museum
where movies on logging are shown. Take the exit on
4th, turn right, and walk to SW Madison. From here,
turn right and cross SW 5th. On your right is the Standard Plaza and a cast bronze "Ring of Time" (17). At
SW 6th, turn left to SW Columbia, and left again. The
Equitable Center (18), and the 40-story First National
Bank Tower (19), Portland's tallest building, will be on
your left side. Refresh yourself with a fantastic view of
the Willamette River from the cafe on the 28th floor.

Return to ground level and continue walking on SW
Columbia to SW 3rd. At SW 3rd, walk left for a block
to the Schrunk Plaza (20) or turn right on SW 3rd and
head back to your point of departure.

For further information, contact Portland Walking
Tours, P.O. Box 4322, Portland, OR 97208; or Portland Chamber of Commerce, 824 SW 5th Ave., Portland, OR 97204.

Quebec City, Quebec
Canada

Old Quebec. An area steeped in history and French lore, Old Quebec covers approximately four square miles. It has two sections, an Upper and a Lower town. The world famous Citadel (old fort) towers 347 feet above the southwest part of town. It is the highest point on the seven-mile-long Cape Diamond.

North of the Citadel is Upper Town, encircled in part by a stone wall. The wall is about 35 feet high and has three gates. Most of Quebec's best hotels, shops, monuments, parks, restaurants, colleges and parliament buildings are in this section.

From the Citadel to the famous hotel, Chateau Frontenac, is a 60-foot wide walkway along the cliffs. From this walkway you have an excellent view of the town of Levis across the St. Lawrence River.

Northeast of Upper Town is Lower Town. It includes most of the business and industrial districts of Quebec. Only a few feet above sea level, it's located on a narrow strip of land between the St. Lawrence and St. Charles rivers. Some of the oldest and narrowest streets in the city—a few only eight feet wide—are in this area. Two in particular are Sous le Cap and Champlain. Notre Dame des Victoires church is located on the site of the log cabin of Samuel de Champlain, the French explorer. The best-known landmark in this area is a square called Place Royale.

Quebec has about 350 acres of parks. A few are Exposition Park, Victorian Park, Cartier-Brebeuf Park, and Battlefields Park which includes the historic Plains of Abraham. Of interest to almost everyone is that six and a half miles north of Quebec are the 274-foot Montmorency Falls.

Contact the Quebec Tourism and Convention Bureau, 60 Rue d'Auteuil, Quebec City, Quebec, Canada G1R 4M8 for a summary of Old Quebec walking tours.

San Diego, California

Parks. San Diego has about 120 of them. Mission Bay Park is the largest. It covers 4,200 acres. The park includes Mission Bay, the Pacific Coast, miles of beach area, and Sea World. Balboa Park, in the center of the city, comprises 1,400 acres.

You can also try the beaches at Coronado, Rosecrans Street to Cabrillo Monument Drive, and then to the Cabrillo Monument itself along the ocean.

For further information, contact San Diego Chamber of Commerce, 223 A St., Suite 300, San Diego, CA 92101.

San Francisco, California

San Francisco Tours. San Francisco is The Place to walk. But beware, its hills can drain you. Start off on the level on Embarcadero at the northeast corner of the city. Embarcadero runs parallel to the waterfront. Here, you can get a good look at the ships from many countries. At the north end of the waterfront is the famous Fisherman's Wharf with its shops, restaurants, and interesting sights. Watch for the small fishing boats coming in with loads of fish and crabs.

Moored at Fisherman's Wharf is the *Balclutha,* a three-masted sailing ship that rounded Cape Horn during the late 1800s. It is the last ship to have made the dangerous voyage around South America. It is owned by the San Francisco Maritime Museum Association.

From Fisherman's Wharf, take any one of the streets that run south. Walk two blocks until you come to Beach Street. Turn right, and head toward Ghirardelli Square. On your way, you'll pass the cable car turntable. At Ghirardelli Square, you'll find an old chocolate factory which has been converted into shops of all kinds. To the north of Ghirardelli Square is the Maritime Museum where there are preserved relics of ships and the gear of sailors who used to come into the port of San Francisco.

A little farther west is Aquatic Park. Here you can swim in saltwater, fish, or participate in other kinds of outdoor activities. You can end your walk here if you wish or go back to the cable car turntable and pick up the cable car that runs up Hyde Street.

Or you can walk up to Russian Hill. The hill got its name from the nationality of its early residents. Near the top, you'll come to the famous Lombard Street. The street is known for its sharp S-curves, and the flowers and shrubs that line it. Take a walk down Lombard. If you feel up to it, keep walking toward Telegraph Hill just east of Nob and Russian hills. On top of Telegraph Hill is Coit Tower, a shining white memorial to all of San Francisco's firemen. The tower, built in 1933, is 210 feet high. After visiting the tower, turn left on Lombard, then right on Grant toward Chestnut. At Chestnut, turn right and head back to Embarcadero.

For more information, contact Greater San Francisco Chamber of Commerce, 465 California St., 9th Floor, San Francisco, CA 94104.

Seattle, Washington

Waterfront. The Elliot Bay waterfront provides a great place to walk in Seattle. Start your tour at the Port of Seattle to the north and stroll south along the Alaskan Way, with the water to your right, until you come to the Harbor Patrol Station at the south end. Along the way are many historic points of interest.

For further information, contact the Department of Community Development, 400 Yesler Ave., Suite 300, Seattle, WA 98101. Also contact King County Department of Planning and Community Development Parks Division, West 226 King County Courthouse, 516 3rd Ave., Seattle, WA 98104.

Vancouver, British Columbia
Canada

Gastown-Chinatown. For an understanding of how Vancouver began, start at West Cordova Street near where the Sea Bus sails from North Vancouver across the Burrard Inlet. Granville Square (1) is in front of you. Walk east. On your left is the Canadian-Pacific Rail Station (2). On the right, between Seymore and Richards, is Harbor Center (3) which includes an office tower over 450 feet high. Turn onto Water Street. In the 100 block, you will come to Gaslight Square (4) with its shops, restaurants, stores, and nightclubs done up with antique charm.

Farther along Water Street is the Garage (5). Walk through the courtyard to Blood Alley Square (6). At West Cordova Street, turn left. On your right is the Dunn Miller Block (7). This was Vancouver's first lending library and the site of the first public Jewish services in the city.

At Carrall Street, go right (south) to enter Chinatown (8). At the corner of Pender and Carrall is the Chinese Free Mason's Building (9). At Eight West Pender is the Sam Kee Building (10). To the west of

---

Vancouver—Map Legend

Start

(1) Granville Square	(11) Chinese Cultural Center
(2) Canadian-Pacific Rail Station	(12) Chinese Times
	(13) Wong's Benevolent Society
(3) Harbor Center	(14) Bank of Montreal
(4) Gaslight Square	(15) Tai Hing Bldg.
(5) Garage	(16) Kuomintang Bldg.
(6) Blood Alley Square	(17) Carnegie Library
(7) Dunn Miller Block	(18) Law Courts
(8) Chinatown	(19) Fire Hall #8
(9) Chinese Free Mason's Bldg.	(20) Hotel Europe
(10) Sam Kee Bldg.	(21) Maple Tree Square

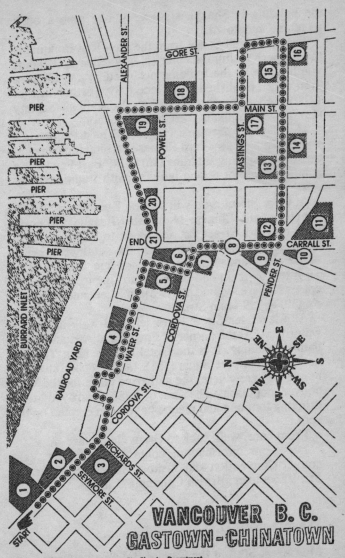

Used by permission of the Vancouver City Planning Department

the building is Shanghai Alley, at one time a busy street in Chinatown.

Across Carrall Street from the Sam Kee Building is the Chinese Cultural Center (11). Walking up Pender, you'll come to the building occupied by the *Chinese Times* (12), published here since 1939. Farther east (at 121-125 East Pender) is Wong's Benevolent Society (13). It was originally the Chinese School.

The Bank of Montreal (14) at 178 East Pender is a good example of modern Chinese architecture. In contrast, the Tai Hing Building (15) at 249 East Pender is a good example of a new building with traditional features.

At Gore Street, you will see the Kuomintang Building (16) of the Chinese Nationalist League. Go north (left) on Gore Street for one block to Hastings. Turn left again and walk to Main. On the southwest corner of Hastings and Main is the Carnegie Library (17). Turn left on main and walk toward the inlet. The law courts (18) are located at 222 Main Street and Fire Hall #8 (19) at 199 Main Street.

At Alexander Street, turn left and walk along the waterfront. At the corner of Powell and Alexander is a flatiron building. It is the Hotel Europe (20). You are now at Maple Tree Square (21). In the 1800s, a leaning maple tree grew here, the gathering place for the Vancouver populace. The fire of 1886 destroyed it. A drinking fountain and plaque have been erected on the spot.

From here, walk back to Granville Square.

For more information, contact the Greater Vancouver Convention and Visitors Bureau, 650 Burrard St., Vancouver, British Columbia, Canada.

Washington, D.C.

Mall Area. Start at the Capitol Building between Constitution and Independence avenues. Walk west on

Pennsylvania Avenue. Just before it intersects with Constitution, you'll see the National Gallery of Art East (1) on your left-hand side. Turn left on Constitution Avenue. On your left, you'll find the main building of the National Gallery of Art (2). Walk along Constitution and past 9th Street; you'll see the Museum of Natural History (3) on your left. On your right is the Justice Department (4) and the Internal Revenue Service (5). Farther on is the Museum of Natural History and Technology (6) and on your right is the Labor Department (7). Any one of these would be a fascinating stop—now or another day.

At 15th Street, turn right and proceed north. On the left is the Ellipse of the White House grounds (8) and on your right, the Commerce Department (9). Walk up 15th Street to Pennsylvania Avenue. To your left will be the Treasury Department (10). Turn left on Pennsylvania Avenue. The White House is on your left (11) and Lafayette Park (12) on your right. At 17th Street, turn left and walk south. You will pass the Executive Office to the left (13) and, farther on down, Corcoran Art Gallery (14) on your right. The Red Cross Building (15) and Constitution Mall (16) are a short distance down on the same side.

At Constitution Avenue, swing left into the park toward the Washington Monument (17). Return to Constitution and walk west along the Constitution Gardens (18). As you walk, you'll pass the Bureau of Indian Affairs (19), the Federal Reserve Building (20), and the National Academy of Sciences (21). At 23rd, turn left for a look at the Lincoln Memorial (22). You are now in West Potomac Park. After a visit to the memorial, walk south to Independence Avenue, turn to your left and walk down toward the Tidal Basin (23). Continue east on Independence past 14th Street where you will find the Agriculture Department (24) and the Forrestal Building (25) on the right and the Smithsonian Institution (26) on your left. Farther along Independence Avenue, just before you reach Maryland Avenue, you

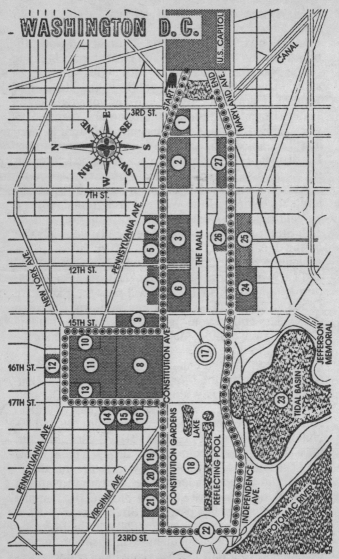

Used by permission of the District of Columbia Dept. of Transportation

Washington—Map Legend

Start-Capitol Bldg.

 (1) National Gallery of Art
      East
 (2) National Gallery of Art
 (3) Museum of Natural History
 (4) Justice Department
 (5) Internal Revenue Service
 (6) Museum of Natural History
      and Technology
 (7) Labor Department
 (8) White House Ellipse
 (9) Commerce Department
(10) Treasury Department
(11) White House
(12) Lafayette Park
(13) Executive Office
(14) Corcoran Art Gallery

(15) Red Cross Bldg.
(16) Constitution Mall
(17) Washington Monument
(18) Constitution Gardens
(19) Bureau of Indian Affairs
(20) Federal Reserve Bldg.
(21) National Academy of
      Sciences
(22) Lincoln Memorial
(23) Tidal Basin
(24) Agriculture Department
(25) Forrestal Bldg.
(26) Smithsonian Institution
(27) National Air and Space
      Museum

---

will pass the National Air and Space Museum (27) on your left. Make an oblique left onto Maryland Avenue and head back to the Capitol. On your right, you'll find the Botanic Gardens. There's a lot to see along this two and a quarter mile long mall.

For further information, contact the District of Columbia Chamber of Commerce, Inc., 1319 F Street, NW, (9th Floor), Washington, D.C. 20004.

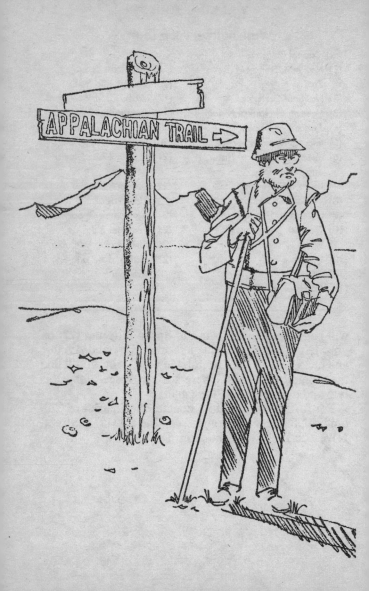

FEATS OF WALKING

MEET THE WALKERS WHO'VE EARNED A PLACE IN THE RECORD BOOKS.

"Take it easy," we've said. "Don't overextend yourself." "Walk without pain." That's good advice. We've heard of a lot of people who've ignored this advice, and what did it get them?

It got them a place in the record books. Competition seems to be a human instinct. Regardless of the endeavor, some people have the urge to do it the fastest, the longest, the best, even the worst, on record. Walking is no different.

One of the more unusual feats of walking was combined with fasting. On June 1, 1926, George Hassler Johnson set out to walk from Chicago to New York without eating anything along the way. Johnson was not a big man: five feet six inches tall; 157 pounds. He wanted to prove that the human body can operate efficiently for long periods of time while subjected to complete fasting.

In his account of the trip, Johnson said he traveled all sorts of roads in all kinds of weather. He was followed by his physician, who checked Johnson's condition daily. He was constantly watched to make sure that he did not have any food with him.

Johnson walked 500 miles and was still going strong as he passed Pittsburgh. However, while approaching the mountains past Greensburg, Pennsylvania, he began to experience difficulty. His feet were sore because most of his body fat had been used to keep his body going, and the bones of his metatarsal arches no longer had pads of fat to cushion them. Nevertheless, Johnson pressed on to the Pennsylvania Mountains. He climbed four and a half miles to the top of the Tuscarora Summit. By the time he arrived in Chambersburg, he had to quit. According to his physician, Johnson was in fine health and good spirits, but his feet were too sore.

What Johnson accomplished on his 20-day walk has never been matched. He covered a total of 577.88 miles—almost 30 miles a day—over rough terrain and primitive highways of the day without eating. After his fasting walk, Johnson regained his weight rapidly, putting on 23 pounds in the first week.

Johnson's walk may sound bizarre to some of you who are just getting started, but once you become hooked on walking, you might find yourself setting all kinds of personal goals.

Those That Make the Record Book

Distance and time—those are what walking records are all about. Some are truly astounding, such as:

Starting out from Singapore on May 4, 1957, David Kwan walked all the way to London in a period of 81 weeks. Averaging 32 miles a day, Kwan passed through 14 countries during his 18,500-mile trek. Plennie L. Wingo covered only 8,000 miles—a mere stroll compared to Kwan's achievement—but Wingo is in the record books because he did his walking in reverse. Wearing special glasses so that he could see where he was going, Wingo started his backward journey in Santa Monica, California, on April 15, 1931; he arrived at his destination—Istanbul, Turkey—on October 24, 1932. As if that were not enough, at age 81,

Wingo decided to celebrate the 45th anniversary of his intercontinental backward walk by walking in reverse from Santa Monica to San Francisco. It took him 85 days to traverse the 452 miles.

Has anyone ever walked around the world? Two brothers, John and David Kunst of Waseca, Minnesota, set out to do precisely that on June 10, 1970. David made it, returning home on October 6, 1974, after covering 14,500 miles. John did not; he was killed by Afghani bandits in 1972.

Distance has been the goal for many walkers, but the competitive types have always been concerned with time as well as mileage. Robert Rinchard of Belgium, for example, holds the record for the annual Strasbourg-to-Paris event. The longest annual contest, it covers 313 to 344 miles. Rinchard set the record in 1974 when he walked 325 miles in 63 hours, 29 minutes.

John Lees of Brighton, England, holds the speed record for walking across the United States. Starting out at Los Angeles City Hall on April 11, 1972, Lees arrived at New York City Hall on June 3, 1972. In other words, he covered 2,876 miles in a period of slightly more than 53 days. Clyde McRae holds the record for crossing Canada. He made it from Halifax to Vancouver—3,764 miles—between May 1 and August 4, 1973.

Then there are the feats in which a walker attempts to cover the greatest distance in a specified amount of time. Jesse Casteneda holds the men's record for distance walked in 24 hours: 142 miles, 448 yards (September 18–19, 1976). Dorothy Whitfield of Bristol, England, holds the women's record for the same time period: 72 miles (October 10–11, 1975). And another Britisher named Lindsay R. Dodd holds the record for the longest distance walking backward in 24 hours: 80 miles (April 9–10, 1976).

Dimitru Dan of Rumania set the record for the 100,000-kilometer (62,137-mile) contest sponsored by the Touring Club de France on April 1, 1910. He set the record because he was the only one of the 200 competitors to finish.

Perhaps the most amazing walking record of them all, though, belongs to Thomas Patrick Benson of Great Britain. Although Benson covered only about 314 miles, he covered that distance without stopping. For nearly 124 consecutive hours (December 19–25, 1975), Benson remained in motion at Moor Park, Preston, England.

The Appalachian Trail

There are all kinds of short-distance and long-distance goals you may want to try to reach some day. But one of them—walking the Appalachian Trail—will give you a sense of history as well as a real sense of accomplishment.

Stretching from Maine to Georgia, the Appalachian Trail originally was a path used by migrating Indians. It was this country's first "interstate" and after the Revolution was maintained by the individual states. As vigorous a walk as it may seem to be, it has been conquered by many avid walkers. Some of the following stories may give you inspiration for your own program.

One of the fastest end-to-end trips on the trail took 70 days. Branley C. Owen, an ex-paratrooper from Knoxville, Tennessee, did it in 1971. On some days he walked as much as 17 hours. He walked without a tent or stove and carried no more than a three-day supply of food. As he walked, he tried to supplement his diet with wild greens and cattail roots. His biggest complaint was that he didn't remember anything about the trip. At last report, he was planning to do it again, only slower. He wants to take in the beauty of the trail.

The first person to hike the entire trail, from Maine to Georgia, in one year was Earl Shaffer of York, Pennsylvania, who did it in 1948. He repeated this feat in 1965, this time in the opposite direction.

Of course, many people do the trail in bits and pieces. Dr. Frederick Luehing of Swarthmore, Pennsylvania, holds the record for taking the most time to finish: it took him 14 years. He was 80 years old when he completed the final 200 miles. He was accompanied along some of those 200 miles by an eight-year-old neighbor, Marc Boyer. Marc has set his own record: he is the youngest person to have completed the entire trail. He completed it by age 13.

The story of Elmer L. Onstott of Ferguson, Missouri, is fascinating. Bob Rodale, editor of *Fitness For Living*, recorded Onstott's trip, which he undertook during the late 1960s. At age 69, Onstott decided to walk the trail non-stop.

He started at Singer Mountain in Georgia in April 1968. He set off on his walking trip in high spirits, seeking adventure, beauty, and the opportunity to take a few photographs. Onstott carried a pack loaded with a small tent, sleeping bag, radio, padded ground cloth, extra clothes, camera, tripod, gadget, bag, food, walking stick, and other equipment. After 150 miles, he sent home the tent, sleeping bag, and radio. But he did carry the rest of the equipment all the way. The gadget bag and tripod were a problem, but he needed them to take pictures. He came to enjoy sleeping on the ground. The only cover he used for the trip was his poncho. Some nights were pretty chilly; yet he didn't catch cold until near the end of the trip.

Those who plan to hike the whole trail—or long stretches of it—often depend on support from someone following them in a car. About every 20 miles, a road intersects the trail, and at those places the hiker can meet his driving partner, pick up some food, and even be taken to a motel to spend the night.

Onstott couldn't arrange automobile support for his adventure. So he worked out a supply plan with his wife. She sent food to specified post offices along the way. Sometimes Onstott would repack the food into smaller parcels and reship it to himself farther up the trail. Occasionally, he would buy food in stores.

Onstott averaged about 12 miles a day. That isn't a fast pace. But his objective was to go slow and enjoy the beauty of nature. On some days, however, he covered as much as 20 miles.

The trail through Virginia and much of the south of the trail had been smoothed out back in the 1930s and is still easy to travel in most places. But north of the Susquehanna River in Pennsylvania, the going can get rough. Onstott fell 30 to 40 times during the trip. And although many of the falls were quite serious, he was never injured badly. He skinned his knee twice, but that was all. One fall, though, brought him close to oblivion. He tried to jump a ledge atop a mountain in Connecticut, and when he landed, his backpack threw him off balance. He went down the trail like a bullet, and ended up lodged between the branches of a little tree growing on the edge of a cliff.

Onstott said, "You don't find sympathy or mercy on the trail. After two to three months, the long walk wears you down. It's a tremendous drain on the human body. A lot of young people fall by the wayside, and don't complete the trip."

During Onstott's trip, he became frightened when he realized he had lost 32 pounds, from 180 to 148. When he looked at his body, he became frightened. He could see every rib sticking out. But he felt he had to keep on going, and he did.

Six months and 10 days after he started, Onstott was one mile from the end of the trail. To finish, he would have to climb up Maine's Mount Katahdin. His health was good, and he still felt strong and vigorous, but a vicious storm made the mountainside unsafe. So after over 190 days of walking, he stopped. He walked the last mile of the Appalachian Trail on another trip early in the fall of 1969. His feat is remarkable for anyone of any age, let alone someone pushing 70.

These record holders demonstrate that there is within all of us the power to do more than we think possible. We only have to try.

REFERENCES

Adams, G. M., and deVries, H. A. "Physiological Effects of an Exercise Training Regimen Upon Women Aged 52 to 79." *Journal of Gerontology* 28 (1973).

Allsen, P. E.; Harrison, J. M.; and Vance, B. *Fitness for Life*. Dubuque, Iowa: William C. Brown, 1976.

Ambrus, L. *Exercise and Emphysema*. Washington, DC: Veteran's Administration Hospital, 1965.

American Medical Association. "Exercise Stress Testing of the Apparently Healthy Individual by Allied Health Personnel." Unpublished statement, November 1974.

————. *Guide to Prescribing Exercise Programs*. Chicago: American Medical Association, 1976.

Anderson, B. *Stretching*. Fullerton, Calif., 1975.

Andrews, V. "The Joy of Jogging." *The New York Times*, December 27, 1976/January 3, 1977.

Aronow, W. S., and Stemmer, E. A. "Two-Year Follow-Up of Angina Pectoris: Medical or Surgical Therapy." *Annals of Internal Medicine*, February 1975.

Asher, W. L. *Treating the Obese*. New York: Medcom Press, 1974.

Astrand, P. O., and Rodahl, K. *Textbook Work Physiology*. New York: McGraw-Hill, 1977.

Barnard, R. J. "The Heart Needs Warm-Up Time." *The Physician and Sportsmedicine*, January 1976.

Bednar, R. "A Dog-Gone Good Way To Exercise." *Fitness for Living*, September/October 1968.

Behnke, A. R., and Wilmore, J. H. *Evaluation and Regulation of Body Build And Composition*. Englewood Cliffs, N.J.: Prentice-Hall, 1974.

Beller, A. S. *Fat and Thin*. New York, N.Y.: Farrar, Straus and Giroux, 1977.

Beloc, N. D. "The Relationship of Health Practices and Mortality." *Preventive Medicine* 2 (1973).

Benson, H. *The Relaxation Response*. New York: William Morrow, 1975.

Bingham, D. "Walk Away From Leg Pain." *Fitness for Living,* September/October 1971.

Brinkman, G. "They Do It By the Millions!" *Fitness For Living*. July/August 1969.

Brock, T. "Let's Take A Nice Brisk Walk." *Fitness For Living*. January/February 1968.

Brody, J. E. "Jogging Is Like a Drug: Watch the Dosage, Beware the Problems." *The New York Times,* November 10, 1976.

Brunner, D. "The Influence of Physical Activity on Incidence and Prognosis of Ischemic Heart Disease." In Raab, Wilhelm, (ed.), *Prevention of Ischemic Heart Disease, Principles and Practice*. Springfield, Ill.: Charles C. Thomas, 1966.

Bucher, C. A. "Exercise Is 'Plain Good Business.'" *Reader's Digest,* Feb. '76.

Cantwell, J. D. "Athletes' Hearts: Disease and Nondisease." *The Physician and Sportsmedicine,* September 1973.

Claremont, A., and Bostian, L. "Where Do You Begin?" *Runner's World,* September 1976.

Conniff, J. C. G. "Getting On A Good Footing," *The New York Times Magazine,* April 23, 1978.

Conrad, C. C. "How Different Sports Rate in Promoting Physical Fitness." *Medical Times,* May 1976.

Consumer Guide Magazine, eds. *The Running Book*. Skokie, Ill.: Publications International, 1978.

Cooper, K. H. *Aerobics*. New York: Bantam Books, 1968.

———. *The New Aerobics*. New York: Bantam Books, 1970.

———. *Aerobics for Women*. New York: Bantam Books, 1972.

———. *The Aerobics Way.* New York: M. Evans and Co., 1977.

Cooter, G. R. et al. "Do Long Hair and Football Uniforms Impair Heat Loss?" *The Physician and Sportsmedicine,* February 1975.

Corday, E. "Status of Coronary Bypass Surgery." *Journal of the American Medical Association,* March 24, 1975.

DeVries, H. A. "Exercise Intensity Threshold for Improvement of Cardiovascular-Respiratory Function in Older Men." *Geriatrics,* April 1971.

———. "Physiological Effects of an Exercise Training Regimen Upon Men Aged 52–88." *Journal of Gerontology* 25 (1970).

———. *Vigor Regained.* Englewood Cliffs, N.J.: Prentice-Hall, 1974.

———. "Prescription of Exercise for Older Men from Telemetered Exercise Heart Rate Data." Unpublished, undated paper.

DeVries, H. A., and Adams, G. M. "Comparison of Exercise Responses in Old and Young Men: I. The Cardiac Effort/Total Body Effort Relationship." *Journal of Gerontology* 27 (1972).

———. "Electromyographic Comparison of Single Doses of Exercise and Meprobamate as to the Effects on Muscular Relaxation." *American Journal of Physical Medicine* 51 (1972).

Ducroquet, R.; Ducroquet, J.; and Ducroquet, P. *Walking and Limping.* Philadelphia: J. B. Lippincott, 1968.

Dutton, R. E. "The Executive and Physical Fitness." *Personnel Administration,* March/April 1966.

Ediger, D. "Charting Body Heat—in Color." *The Physician and Sportsmedicine,* January 1975.

Elrick, H., et al. "Indians Who Run 100 Miles on 15,000 Calories a Day." *The Physician and Sportsmedicine,* February 1976.

"Fitness Movement Seen Curbing High Cost of Illness to U.S. Industry." *Commerce Today,* February 3, 1975.

Fixx, J. F. *The Complete Book of Running.* New York: Random House, 1977.

Fletcher, C. *The New Complete Walker*. New York: Alfred A. Knopf, 1977.

Foss, M. L., et al. "Initial Work Tolerance of Extremely Obese Patients." *Archives of Physical Medicine and Rehabilitation*, February 1975.

Furlong, W. B. "The Fun in Fun." *Psychology Today*, June 1976.

Giguere, P. "Boston Marathon—Beating the Heat with Common Sense and Water." *The Physician and Sportsmedicine*, June 1976.

Glasser, W. *Positive Addiction*. New York: Harper and Row, 1976.

Glover, B. and Shephard, J. *The Runner's Handbook*. NY: Viking Press, 1978.

Golding, L. A. "Effects of Physical Training Upon Total Serum Cholesterol Levels." *Research Quarterly*, December 1961.

Goldstein, J. "Walkers of the World, Unite!" *Fitness For Living*, May/June 1968.

Gwinup, G. "Effect of Exercise Alone on the Weight of Obese Women." *Archives of Internal Medicine*, May 1975.

Haberern, J. "The Fitness Finders Arrive." *Fitness For Living*, July/August 1970.

Hanrahan, P. "Smile and Drive Them Crazy." *Runner's World*, October 1976.

Harger, B. S., et al. "The Caloric Cost of Running." *Journal of the American Medical Association*, April 22, 1974.

Haskell, W., et al. "Plasma Lipids and Lipoproteins in Women Runners." Presented to American Heart Association, November 1975.

"Health Practices and Physical Health Status." *Physical Fitness Research Digest*, April 1976.

"Heat Peril In Distance Runs Spurs ACSM Guideline Alert." *The Physician and Sportsmedicine*, July 1975.

Hellerstein, H. "Exploring the Effects of Exercise on Hypertension." *The Physician and Sportsmedicine*, December 1976.

Henderson, J. *Long Slow Distance: The Humane Way To Train*. Mountain View, Calif.: World Publications, 1969.

———. "New Beginnings in Running." *Runner's World*, April 1976.

———. *Run Gently, Run Long*. Mountain View, Calif.: World Publications, 1974.

———. "The Six in Ten Who Break Down," *Runner's World*, Dec. 1975.

Higdon, H. *Fitness After Forty*. Mountain View, CA: World Publications '77.

Hlavac, H. F. *The Foot Book*. Mountain View, CA: World Publications, '77.

Hocking, J. H. "Do You Know How To Walk?" *Recreation*, May 1942.

"How To Get Fit? Just Put One Foot After Another." *Executive Fitness Newsletter*, February 25, 1978.

Howorth, M. D. "The Art and Technique of Walking." *Consumer Bulletin*, April 1973.

Illich, I., and Keen, S., "Medicine Is a Major Threat to Health." *Psychology Today*, May 1976.

Intercollege Research, eds. "Exercise: A Heartening Life-Lengthener?" *Intercollege Research*, Pennsylvania State University, January 1976.

Jackson, D. W., and Bailey, D. "Shin Splints in the Young Athlete: A Nonspecific Diagnosis." *The Physician and Sportsmedicine*, March 1975.

The Jogger, eds. "Harry Hlavac, Jogging Podiatrist." *The Jogger*, July/Aug. '76.

Kasch, F. W. "The Effects of Exercise on the Aging Process." *The Physician and Sportsmedicine*, June 1976.

———. "The Energy Cost of Walking and Hiking." *The Physician and Sportsmedicine*, July 1976.

———. "Physiological Variables During Ten Years of Endurance Exercise." *Medicine and Science in Sports* 8 (1976).

Kasch, F. W., et al. "Cardiovascular Changes in Middle-Aged Men During Two Years of Training." *Journal of Applied Physiology*, January 1973.

Katch, F. I., and McArdle, W. D. *Nutrition, Weight Control, and Exercise*. Boston, Mass.: Houghton, Mifflin, 1977.

Kavanagh, T. "A Conditioning Programme for the Elderly." *Canadian Family Physician*, July 1971.

———. *Heart Attack? Counterattack!* Toronto: Van Nostrand Reinhold, 1976.

"Keeping Fit in the Company Gym." *Fortune,* October 1975.

Kiell, P. J. and Frelinghuysen, J. S. *Keep Your Heart Running*. New York: Winchester Press, 1976.

King, S. "United States Plans To Turn Old Rail Beds Into Recreation Trails." *The New York Times*, May 3, 1978.

Klaw, S. *The Great American Medical Show: The Unhealthy State of U.S. Medical Care and What Can be Done About It*. NY: Viking Press, '75.

Knowles, J. "Wiser Way of Living, Not Dramatic Cures Seen as Key to Health. Preventive Care to Become More Important." *Wall Street Journal*, 3/23/76.

Konecke, S. P. "Joggers' Foot and Leg Problems Can Be Helped." *The Jogger,* July/August 1976.

Kostrubala, T. *The Joy of Running*. Philadelphia: J. P. Lippincott, 1976.

Kuntzleman, C. *Activetics*. New York: Peter H. Wyden, 1975.

———. "Are Your Hormones Killing You?" *Fitness For Living,* November/December, 1970.

———. *Concepts In Health and Fitness*. Spring Arbor, Mich.: Arbor Press, 1978.

———. *The Exerciser's Handbook*. New York: David McKay, 1978.

———. *The Physical Fitness Encyclopedia*. Emmaus, Penn.: Rodale Books, 1970.

Kuntzleman, C.; and *Consumer Guide Magazine*, eds. *Rating The Exercises*. New York: William Morrow and Co., 1978.

Lake, A. "How Much Good Does Exercise Do You?" *Woman's Day,* Oct. '75.

Lance, K. *Running For Health and Beauty*. New York: Bobbs-Merril, 1977.

Lawrence, R. M. "Race Walking for Everyone." *Today's Jogger,* March 1978.

Leonard, G. *The Ultimate Athlete*. New York: Viking Press, 1975.

———. "The Holistic Health Revolution." *New West,* May 10, 1976.

Lewis, S., et al. "Effects of Physical Activity on Weight Reduction in Obese Middle Aged Women." *The American Journal of Clinical Nutrition* 29 (1976).

Lilliefors, J. "The Need to Fail." *Runner's World,* April 1976.

———. "Training the Head." *Runner's World,* May 1976.

Loeschhorn, J. "Running Shoes." *WomenSports,* February 1976.

Lopez, S., et al. "Effect of Exercise and Physical Fitness on Serum Lipids and Lipoproteins." *Atherosclerosis* 20 (1974).

Luria, M. H., and Koepke, K. R. "The Physical Conditioning Effects of Walking." *Journal of Sports Medicine* 15 (1975).

McCormick, L. "Race Walker's Stride a Lonely Course In The United States." *Christian Science Monitor,* June 18, 1973.

McDermott, B. "Going Through Life at a Walk." *Sports Illustrated.* 5/8/78.

McGregor, M. "The Coronary Collateral Circulation." *Circulation,* Oct. 1975.

McWhirter, N. *Guinness Book of World Records,* New York: Bantam Books, 1977.

"Man Called Prone to Extinction if Not Encouraged to Walk More." *Medical Tribune,* June 30, 1971.

Mahoney, M. J., and Mahoney, K. "Fight Fat with Behavior Control." *Psychology Today,* May 1976.

Mayes, D. S. "What's Round and Pounds the Ground? A Slogger!" *The Physician and Sportsmedicine,* April 1976.

"May Your Hearts Be Ever Young and Gay." *Executive Health* 10 (1973).

Menier, D. R., and Pugh, L. G. C. E. "The Relation of Oxygen Intake and Velocity of Walking and Running in Competition Walkers." *Journal of Physiology* 197 (1968).

Michener, J. A. *Sports in America*. New York: Random House, 1976.

Miller, B. F., and Galton, L. *Freedom from Heart Attacks*. New York: Simon and Schuster, 1972.

Miller, G. J., and Miller, N. E., "Plasma-High-Density-Lipoprotein Concentration and Development of Ischaemic Heart-Disease." *Lancet,* 1/4/75.

Milne, L. J., and Milne, M. *The Mountains*. New York: Time, 1962.

Mirkin, G. "A Key to Bad Knee Is a Fault in the Foot." *Washington Post,* June 17, 1976.

———. "Why Every Athlete Needs Muscle-Stretching Exercises." *Washington Post,* April 1, 1976.

———. "How Much Training Do You Need?" *Washington Post,* 6/3/76.

Mundth, E. D., and Austen, W. G. "Surgical Measures for Coronary Heart Disease." *New England Journal of Medicine,* July 3, 1975; July 10, 1975; and July 17, 1975.

Myers, C. R. "The Nationwide YMCA Cardiovascular Health Program." *Journal of Physical Education,* Summer 1976.

———. *The YMCA Physical Fitness Handbook*. New York: Popular Library, 1975.

Myers, C. R.; Golding, L.; and Sinning, W. eds. *The Y's Way To Physical Fitness*. Emmaus, Penn.: Rodale Press, 1973.

Napier, J. "The Antiquity of Human Walking." *Scientific American,* April 1967.

"National Adult Physical Fitness Survey." *The President's Council on Physical Fitness and Sports Newsletter,* May 1973.

National Geographic Society. *Wilderness U.S.A*. Washington, D.C.: National Geographic Society, 1973.

National Wildlife Federation. *Conservation Directory*. Washington, D.C.: The National Wildlife Federation, 1978.

Naughton, J., and Nagle, F. "Peak Oxygen Intake During Physical Fitness Program for Middle-Aged Men." *Journal of the American Medical Association*, March 15, 1965.

Nelson, C. M. "Rehabilitation Emphasis Should Be On Exercise." *The Physician and Sportsmedicine*, September 1976.

"New Rx For A Healthier Heart: 2,000 Calories of Sweat a Week." *Executive Fitness Newsletter*, January 14, 1978.

Norman, J. "The Tarahumaras: Mexico's Long Distance Runners." *National Geographic*, May 1976.

"On Walking . . . Nature's Own Amazing 'Anti-Age Antibiotic.'" *Executive Health* 14 (1978).

Overbeke, J. E. "Can Health Care Costs be Tamed?" *Industry Week*, 5/3/76.

Paffenberger, R. S., Jr.; and Hale, W. E. "Work Activity and Coronary Heart Mortality." *New England Journal of Medicine*, March 13, 1975.

Paul, L. "Sport Is A Three-Letter Word." *Intellectual Digest*, June 1974.

Pearson, K. "The Control of Walking." *Scientific American*, December 1976.

The Physician and Sportsmedicine, eds. "Achilles Tendon Problems Increase," *The Physician and Sportsmedicine*, March 1976.

———. "Balancing Heat Stress, Fluids, and Electrolytes." *The Physician and Sportsmedicine*, August, 1975.

———. "Exercise and the Heart." *The Physician and Sportsmedicine*, March 1974.

———. "Exercise Prescription Guidelines Listed." *The Physician and Sportsmedicine*, July 1975.

———. "Foot Problems in Runners." *The Physician and Sportsmedicine*, July 1976.

———. "Overcoming Overprotection of the Elderly." *The Physician and Sportsmedicine*, June 1976.

———. "Roger Bannister: 'Human Beings Are Not The Same.'" *The Physician and Sportsmedicine*, September 1974.

———. "What to Cover in Office Evaluation for Exercise." *The Physician and Sportsmedicine*, June 1976.

"Pitcher Who Sets Two Records After MI Gets Heart Award." *Medical Tribune,* May 15, 1974.

Pollock, M. L. "How Much Exercise is Enough?" *The Physician and Sportsmedicine,* June 1978.

Pollock, M. L., et al. "Effects of Walking on Body Composition and Cardiovascular Function of Middle Aged Men." *Journal of Applied Physiology,* January 1971.

————. "Physiologic Responses of Men 49 to 65 Years of Age to Endurance Training." *American Geriatrics Society,* March 1976.

Pollock, M. L.; Wilmore, J. H.; and Fox, S. M. *Health and Fitness Through Physical Activity:* New York: John Wiley and Sons, 1978.

The President's Council on Physical Fitness and Sports. "Exercise and Weight Control." Washington, D.C.: Superintendent of Documents, United States Government Printing Office.

Pugh, L. G. C. E. "The Influence of Wind Resistance in Running and Walking and the Mechanical Efficiency of Work Against Horizontal or Vertical Forces." *Journal of Physiology* 213 (1971).

Rarick, G. L. *Physical Activity: Human Growth and Development.* New York: Academic Press, 1973.

Reed, R. "Going Walk-About in a Jumbo Jet." *Times of London,* July 17, 1976.

Renold, A. E., and Gahill, G. F. *Adipose Tissue.* Washington, D.C.: American Physiological Society, 1965.

Rinehart, L. M. "Exercise: The Key to a Healthy Old Age." *Fitness For Living,* July/August 1973.

Rodale, R. "Walk Before You Run." *Fitness For Living,* May/June 1969.

————. "Take a Long Walk!" *Fitness For Living,* March/April 1969.

Rose, C. L., and Cohen, M. L. "Relative Importance of Physical Activity for Longevity." Unpublished report of a study conducted at Veterans Administration Outpatient Clinic, Boston.

Rudner, R. *Off and Walking.* New York: Holt, Rinehart, and Winston, 1977.

Ruffer, W. A. "A Study of Extreme Physical Activity Groups of Young Men." *Research Quarterly,* May 1965.

Runner's World, eds. "The 1979 Runner's World Shoe Survey." *Runner's World,* October 1978.

Ryan, A. J. "Aging, Exercise, and Longevity." *The Physician and Sportsmedicine,* June 1975.

————. "Carotid Palpation Practice Questioned." *The Physician and Sportsmedicine,* September 1976.

————. "Heat Stress and the Vulnerable Athlete." *The Physician and Sportsmedicine,* June 1973.

Ryan, A. J.; and Allman, F. L., Jr. *Sports Medicine,* New York: Academic Press, 1974.

Ryan, A. J.; Dempsey, J. A.; Gordon, E. S.; Foss, M. L.; and Oscai, L. D. "Charting the Factors of Fatness: A Round Table." *The Physician and Sportsmedicine,* July 1975.

Seder, J. I. "Heel Injuries Incurred in Running and Jumping." *The Physician and Sportsmedicine,* October 1976.

Seyle, H. "Stress." *Intellectual Digest,* June 1974.

————. *Stress Without Distress.* Philadelphia: J. P. Lippincott, Inc.

————. The Stress of Life. New York: McGraw-Hill, 1956.

Sheehan, G. "Come and Play." *The Physician and Sportsmedicine,* Nov. 1974.

————. "Let Me Do My Thing—And You Can Do Yours." *The Physician and Sportsmedicine,* June 1975.

————. "Let's Hear It for Morton's Foot." *The Physician and Sportsmedicine,* March 1974.

————. *Running and Being: "The Total Experience."* New York: Simon and Schuster, 1978.

Stamford, B. A.; Hambacher, W.; and Fallica, A. "Effects of Daily Physical Exercise on the Psychiatric State of Institutionalized Geriatric Mental Patients." *The Research Quarterly,* March 1974.

Stone, F. "Stay in Shape for the Rigors of Management '75: 1. A Sound Mind . . ." *Management Review,* January 1975.

Sussman, A., and Goode, R. *The Magic of Walking.* New York: Simon and Schuster, 1967.

"The Fitness Mania." *U.S. News and World Report*, 2/27/78.

Thomas, C. T. "Help For Tired, Aching Legs." *Fitness For Living*, November/December 1971.

Thomson, P. "Fifty-Five Men, Women, and Grandfathers Have Hiked All 2,025 Miles of the Appalachian Trail." *The New York Times*, May 9, 1971.

Tossetti, J. "Tips on Dealing with Lightning on the Links." *The Physician and Sportsmedicine*, May 1976.

Turner, R., and Ball, K. "The Cardiologist's Responsibility for Preventing Coronary Heart Disease." *American Heart Journal*, February 1976.

Van Aaken, E. *The Van Aaken Method*, Mountain View, Calif.: World Publications, 1976.

Van Dyck, D. "Big Brother Wants You To Take A Walk!" *Detroit Free Press*, July 12, 1978.

"Walk Away From Emphysema." *Fitness For Living*, Sept./Oct. 1969.

Watts, M. T., "The Story of a Single Footpath." *Fitness For Living*, September/October 1968.

White, J. R., and Hunt, H. F. "When Doctors Test Themselves, the Prescription is Exercise." *The Physician and Sportsmedicine*, December 1975.

"Will Exercise Improve Your Production?" *Pilot's Log*. New England Mutual Life Insurance Company, September 1976.

Wilmore, J. *Exercise And Science Reviews*. New York: Academic Press (assorted volumes).

Wilson, N. L., ed. *Obesity*. Philadelphia: F. A. Davis, 1969.

Wood, P. D. "Bos(huff)ton(puff)or(sigh) Bust." *The New York Times*, 4/21/75.

———. "Concentrations of Plasma Lipids and Lipoproteins in Male and Female Long-Distance Runners." Paper presented at International Congress of Physical Activity Sciences, Quebec, 1976.

INDEX

A

B

H

J

K

L

M